DE-STRESS YOUR LIFE: TURN CHAOS INTO CALM

Easy, Sustainable Steps to Lifestyle Rituals
that Drain Stress and Generate Energy and Calm

DEBORAH RANKIN, MS, RDN

De-Stress Your Life: Turn Chaos Into Calm

Easy, Sustainable Steps to Lifestyle Rituals That Drain Stress and Generate Energy and Calm

The publisher and author of this book have made reasonable efforts to ensure that the information contained herein is accurate, but no warranty is provided nor results guaranteed. In authoring and publishing this book, neither the author nor the publisher is rendering legal, medical, or other professional services. If medical or other expert assistance is required, please consult with your primary care provider or another competent professional.

ISBN 978-1-7358972-0-2 (print)
978-1-7358972-1-9 (eBook)

Published by:
Healthy Habits Communications LLC
Arvada, CO

Contents

Foreword

PUT YOUR OWN OXYGEN MASK ON FIRST, BEFORE ASSISTING OTHERS.

—every flight attendant on every airplane

This book will help you discover and implement an exciting truth: when you take care of yourself, life is easier. You enjoy what you do, and you have energy and presence to share abundantly with those around you.

The opposite is also true. When you neglect your needs and push yourself to the limit for days, weeks, and months, you risk an advanced state of depression and exhaustion known as burnout. Entrepreneurs, small business owners, and creative artists are prone to burnout because of the long hours and intense pace at which they work, compounded by their great personal responsibility and passion. Passion—the juice that drives great achievement and innovation—also makes burnout more likely because those with passion care so much about how things turn out.

I expect you are reading this book because you want to be healthy. Have you asked yourself why health is important to you? Do you want to live longer? Or do you hope to achieve certain numbers (for example, bench press a certain weight, complete a distance event in a certain time, or better your LDL cholesterol, blood sugar, or blood pressure)? Are you motivated to lose weight for an appearance you feel will make you more attractive to others? These are all respectable, worthwhile goals. But let us look deeper.

What's so great about living longer, if it's not a meaningful, satisfying life?

> *The important thing to you is not*
> *how many years in your life, but*
> *how much life in your years!*
>
> *—advertising quote in the 1947 Chicago Daily Tribune*

Numbers such as strength, speed, cholesterol, blood sugar, blood pressure, and weight are important. What then? What kind of life do you live with your good numbers?

Chances are, you are already attractive enough. I know people of all weights and shapes who are in loving relationships. I also know thin, fit people who feel lonely and unattached. It is easy to judge yourself according to images from advertising and social media and conclude that eat less or exercise more + lose weight = be happier. Yet evidence suggests that close friends, strong social connections, and meaningful work contribute more to your health and happiness than an arbitrary number on a scale.

When I close my eyes and picture what health and wellness look like for me, here's what I see:

- My friends plan an adventure bike trip to Austria. I am strong and fit enough to go, and enjoy it.
- I chaperone my son's field trip to Boston and tread the Freedom Trail for hours with seven middle-school boys. At the end of the day, I sprint after two escapees with enough speed to catch them, and herd them back to the bus.
- When I visit my three granddaughters, I push their stroller uphill to a park, and then climb the BIG SLIDE. At their house, I can walk up and down a steep flight of stairs a dozen times a day with a twenty-pound toddler in each arm.
- I accept an exciting new job that requires frequent travel. Because I am healthy and strong, I can leave the house at 6:00 a.m., drag a suitcase through several airports, stand all day at a trade show, meet clients for dinner, then get up the next day and do it all over again.
- I rely on stress-reducing strategies, support of friends, and journaling to balance my emotions as I settle complex affairs after my father's death. This helps my siblings, and keeps our family intact.

My goal is to help you to discover and internalize one thing from reading this book: a healthy lifestyle is not a curse or punishment you must endure.

Rather, it is a wellspring of pleasant energy, deep peace, and rich experience that makes all parts of your life more satisfying and meaningful.

I decided to write *De-Stress Your Life: Turn Chaos Into Calm* after watching clients, friends, and family members I care about take on rigid diet regimes that made them give up whole food groups and follow a difficult, joyless schedule. I saw them spend hard-earned money on supplements and electronic gadgets they used for a while, then abandoned. I noticed they worked so hard they had little energy to enjoy the assets they earned.

I know, based on my personal journey, my training as a registered dietitian nutritionist (RDN) with an advanced degree in nutrition, and my work as a health coach, that there is a better way!

When you eat well, sleep well, and move your body, you tap into a huge reservoir of peace, calmness, and energy. Journaling, deep connections with others, time in nature, and purpose in work release tension and add joy. When you choose healthy habits, your sense of contentment and satisfaction expands. Resilience and a broader perspective cushion you during life's rough patches.

I wrote this book for hard-working, successful people who achieve at work, take care of their family or pets at home, and give time and energy to community organizations. I wrote to people who get it done, for in my career as a registered dietitian and health coach I've noticed that those who go all-out for work and service often neglect to care for themselves. Everything else seems more urgent. Many people set health aside for "when there's time."

I wrote to tell you *this is the time*. You have time now to adopt and maintain small daily changes that will deliver phenomenal gifts like clear thinking, renewed vigor, and a more positive mindset.

Now, take a moment to think about what health means to you. How does a calm and healthy you look and act? See it. Notice details. To define what health means to you, it might help to take a look at my free infographic:

https://stressrelief.deborahrankinrd.com/mywhyforhealth

Write down in this space your why—the reasons you want less stress and more health.

Then if you are able, recline on your back on the floor with your legs extended up a wall. Put your arms out to your sides in a "T" shape. Take five deep breaths, counting to four on both the inhale and the exhale.

Rest. In your mind, watch images of yourself living like the healthy and peaceful self you wrote about above.

Then turn the page and join me in discovering practical strategies that will help you de-stress your life and turn chaos into calm. Together, let's build the behaviors that increase your strength, energy, and joy.

How to Use This Book

Each chapter of this book follows the same format. First, I write about an important health habit and the evidence that shows how and why this behavior is an anchor of good health.

Next comes a discussion of practical tips and strategies. I call this the **Make It Happen** section. Readers of my blog (https://www.deborahrankinrd.com) who answered a survey about what they wanted in this book came out loud and clear in their request for practical how-to ideas. I heard you! This section is here because of you. **Make It Happen** is designed to be a ready reference you can turn to time and again. When you need help or encouragement, flip back to a chapter and find practical ideas to help you get back on track, or a new idea to try. Because I know your life is busy and hectic, **Make It Happen** gives three versions of recommendations, each designed to meet your needs depending on the type of day you are having:

- **A Slammed Day** is one in which you don't have a moment to spare. You rush from one

thing to another and deal with multiple challenges and crises. You put out fires.
- **A Typical Day** has a full schedule, but you manage it well because it's familiar and you know what to expect.
- **A Light Day** is either a day off, or a work day with much flexibility and unscheduled time.

Your life varies, so I provide three variations of practical tips to help you respond to shifting demands with flexibility and creativity.

The third section of each chapter is a personal essay from an accomplished, busy person who faced a challenge in healthy living and dealt with it in a positive way. We are all inspired by real people who face tough challenges. I am honored by the generosity of those who shared their stories so you and I might benefit from their wisdom and experience. Each essay concludes with a brief biographical sketch of the writer, with links or contact information for those you may wish to follow.

The fourth section of each chapter is a blank page titled **Key Take Aways and Action Steps.** I urge you to make the most of this page. The real value of this book depends on what you do with the information you gain. Write down ideas that caught your attention, and commit to an action.

A good format to follow is:

I will do _______ (what) with my ______(how),
starting ____________ (when).

Please use this page. Even though it seems simple, it is quite important. Writing something down leads to deeper thinking and forges a link between ideas and actions. Your brain doesn't have to work so hard to remember an idea if you write it down. Writing something in longhand helps your brain process the concept and prioritize what you act on.

I placed the ten chapters of this book in a sequence built from a foundation of basic health habits that progress toward more complex skills. However, feel free to read the chapters in any order you wish. Because they follow the same general format, each chapter stands on its own. Use this book for inspiration and practical ideas that add healthy habits in your life, one step at a time. In doing so, you will de-stress your life and replace chaos with calm.

Food, Part 1

"ONE CANNOT THINK WELL, LOVE WELL, SLEEP WELL, IF ONE HAS NOT DINED WELL."

—Virginia Woolf in *A Room of One's Own*

One of the first things you learned as a baby was how to feed yourself. Before you could run from danger, get dressed for the day, or use a toilet, you held a bottle or sippy cup between your hands and gulped cool, soothing water or milk. You picked up Cheerios with your thumb and forefinger and put them in your mouth. You kept close to your mother, who offered nourishing breast milk. You made feeding your top priority.

And now, as an adult, what priority do you give to your meals?

Even if you love to eat and struggle with eating too much, it's very likely that you skip breakfast, or grab a sugared coffee concoction from a drive-through on the way to work, lunch on a Diet Coke and packaged peanut butter crackers while you work, then arrive home exhausted and hungry after a long day to face a barren fridge with nothing there for dinner. You might eat take-out for dinner with Netflix for company, or pick up bags of fast food for the family on the way home from soccer practice. You are busy, and there is no time to cook. You decide what to eat as an afterthought, when everything else is done.

One effect of the 2020 COVID-19 pandemic for Americans was a dramatic increase in cooking and eating meals at home. While many people reported they ate healthier meals, others regretted weight gain from stressed-based eating.

If you want to improve your health, feel better, and empower yourself to a more calm and peaceful life, the first and very important step is to re-learn how to nourish yourself with food. You knew how to do this as a baby, for you drank when you were thirsty and made sure you ate when you were hungry. If the big people in your life didn't give you food when you were hungry, you screamed and cried and they soon learned to take care of that for you. If they wanted you to eat when you weren't hungry, you clamped your jaws shut or threw the food on the floor.

Whether you neglect regular meals because you are so busy or struggle with eating more than you may need, one of the most important ideas I want you to embrace as a result of reading this book is that *food is not the enemy.* Food nurtures and supports life, gives strength and energy, helps heal our bodies, and facilitates bonding with others in a spirit of community. Even if you struggle with weight issues, food is not your enemy. Dieting is the enemy, for dieting convinces you to deprive, restrict, and punish yourself.

When I started this book, I went to my public library to see what health and nutrition books were available. I was shocked! A small-town library held two full cases of diet books!

The titles made amazing promises: *Eat this miracle food and lose twenty pounds in three weeks! Do this and drop four sizes without effort! Just cut out these foods and you will never ever be hungry again!*

The world does not need another diet book. You don't need another diet.

If you struggle with weight issues, your past diets may make it harder for you to reach your health and weight goals. This happens in two ways:

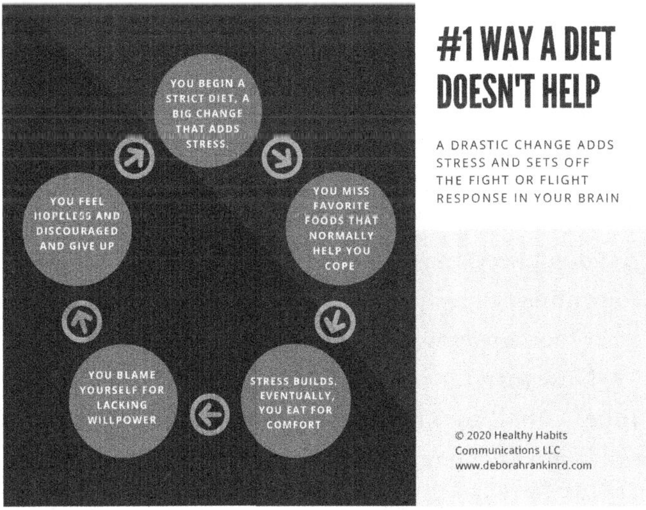

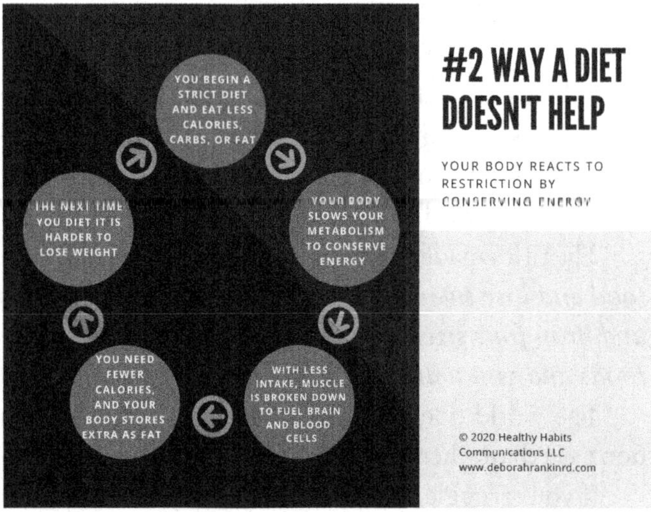

This sounds depressing, but it doesn't have to be. There is a better way. I think it is an easier way. This is the way:

Nourish your body with healthy food. Follow simple practices I'll share so you keep nourishing food in your house and have wholesome things to eat when you are hungry. Lose your cravings with a new mindset that says any food is allowed. Because it is allowed, you don't need to eat it all at once. Act like a baby: feel your hunger. Feel your fullness. Clamp your jaws and push food away when you are not hungry!

Now turn the page to the **Make It Happen** section. Take a small step toward a breakfast habit that helps you begin each day by nourishing your body with food.

Evidence about Food

1. Leidy, H.J., Ortinau, L.C., Douglas, S.M., and Hoertel, H.A. Beneficial Effects of a Higher-Protein Breakfast on the Appetitive, Hormonal, and Neural Signals Controlling Energy Intake Regulation in Overweight/Obese, "Breakfast-Skipping," Late-Adolescent Girls. Am J Clin Nutr. 2013; 97:677–88.
2. Rong, S., Snetselaar, L.G., Xu, G., Sun, Y., Liu, B., Wallace, R.B., and Bao, W. Association of Skipping Breakfast With Cardiovascular and All-Cause Mortality. J Am Coll Cardiol. 2019; 73(16): 2025-2032. DOI: 10.1016/j.jacc.2019.01.065
3. Ruanpeng1, D., Thongprayoon, C., Cheungpasitporn, W., and Harindhanavudhi, T. Sugar and Artificially Sweetened Beverages Linked to Obesity: A Systematic Review and Meta-Analysis. QJM. 2017; 513– 520.
4. Drouin-Chartier, J. P., et al. Changes in Consumption of Sugary Beverages and Artificially Sweetened Beverages and Subsequent Risk of Type 2 Diabetes: Results From Three Large Prospective U.S. Cohorts of Women and Men. Diab Care. 2019; 42(12): 2181-2189.
5. Fowler, S.P.G., Williams, K., and Hazuda, H.P. Diet Soda Intake Is Associated with Long-Term Increases in Waist Circumference in a Bi-Ethnic Cohort of Older Adults: The San Antonio Longitudinal Study of Aging. J Am Geriatr Soc. 2015; 63(4): 708–715.

MAKE IT HAPPEN

Start Each Day by Nourishing Yourself with Food

Breakfast. Do you hate it? Do you eat it? Why or why not?

In the space below, write a sentence or two that describes your thoughts and feelings about breakfast:

Very likely you've heard from parents, teachers, or medical advisors like dietitians that you should eat breakfast.

"It's the most important meal of the day."

"Breakfast revs up your metabolism so you burn more calories the rest of the day."

"You need to eat breakfast so you can concentrate at work/school."

Many people skip breakfast because they need to get a fast start to the day. There *is* ample medical evidence about the benefits of eating breakfast. Would any of the gains listed below be worth shifting your morning routine by twenty minutes?

- People who eat breakfast are less likely to be overweight than those who don't.
- A 2019 study in the *Journal of Cardiology* determined that the risk of death from cardiovascular disease and stroke was 87% higher for Americans who never ate breakfast compared to those who ate breakfast every day. The death rate from all causes was 19% higher for breakfast skippers.
- Weight-loss studies say obese people who eat breakfast lose more weight than those who don't.
- Obese or overweight teenage girls who ate a high-protein breakfast snacked less on high-fat foods in the evenings, and had lower blood levels of a hormone associated with hunger.

While the health benefits of eating breakfast are significant, I believe an even more compelling reason is that it starts each day with the focused intention of taking care of yourself. You work hard, and keep up with a crazy-busy lifestyle. You produce at work, and probably also take care of a dog, cat, child, or elderly parents. Your life can slip by with little attention to the needs of your body.

Breakfast is an essential part of de-stressing your life because it sets an important priority. Eating breakfast says, "I honor myself. I take care of my body first and provide strength and energy for my day." When you eat breakfast, you send a message to yourself that says "I matter. I am here. This is my life and I will live it well."

Although it is vital, breakfast doesn't have to be elaborate or time consuming.

How to Start Every Day

- Drink eight ounces of cold water immediately after you wake up.*
- Enjoy as many cups of unsweetened coffee or tea as you like!**
- Add milk or cream to your coffee or tea if desired.
- Eliminate sugar or artificial sweeteners from your beverages.***

* Drink water first thing in the morning because you are slightly dehydrated when you wake up. Hydrating right away helps you feel alert sooner. Cold water also stimulates your gut. Many people find they avoid constipation

and maintain bowel regularity if they drink cold water in the morning.

** There are health benefits to both coffee and tea. It's great when something we like is good for us!

Coffee improves components of brain function like memory, mood, and reaction times. Research suggests the risk of developing type 2 diabetes is reduced as much as 7% per each daily cup of coffee. Coffee drinkers have up to a 60% lower risk of Parkinson's disease, in addition to less risk of cirrhosis, fatty liver, and liver and colorectal cancer.

Tea may reduce the risk of heart attack and stroke, with up to a 32% reduction in heart attacks reported among those who drank four or more cups of green tea daily. Green tea may also prevent bone loss, and help prevent cavities and tooth loss. Tea contributes antibacterial, antifungal, and anti-inflammatory properties that promote a strong immune system.

*** Avoid sugar in breakfast beverages so you won't get a sugar high followed by a mid-morning crash with tiredness and mental confusion. Intake of both sugary and artificially sweetened beverages is associated with a greater risk of obesity and diabetes. Increased diet soda intake is associated with abdominal obesity. Individuals with chronic headaches who consume large quantities of artificially sweetened beverages on a daily basis might reduce the frequency of their headaches when they eliminate artificial sweeteners.

For a Slammed Day

Grab simple foods and go.

1/4 cup roasted unsalted almonds or peanuts
1 small banana

Pause for a moment as you head to work. If you work from home, step outside. Look at the sky, take a deep breath, and notice how the air feels on your skin. As you eat the simple breakfast, stop once to take a deep breath. Say a silent prayer of thanksgiving for the good things in your life.

For a Typical Day

Enjoy oatmeal jars prepared ahead of time and kept in refrigerator (recipes follow).

To serve, heat in microwave for about two minutes, or until your desired warmth and consistency.

I make three different versions of oatmeal jars and enjoy rotating the unique flavors. You can buy packaged oatmeal cups at the grocery. That is fine, if you like them. Mine cost half as much, don't have added preservatives, keep me full longer, and reduce trash since I re-use the 12-ounce glass jars.

Choco-Nana Oatmeal Jar:

- Drop a half banana in the bottom of a wide-mouth mason jar.
- Mash in 1/2 teaspoon cocoa power.
- Add 1/4 cup steel-cut organic oats* and 3/4 cup milk.
- Dab one teaspoon peanut butter on top.
- Seal and refrigerate overnight. Can keep 2-3 nights in fridge.

Berry Delicious Oatmeal Jar:

- Put 1/4 cup steel-cut organic oats* in a wide-mouth mason jar.
- Pour in 3/4 cup milk.
- Top with 1/4 cup walnut halves and 1-2 Tablespoons frozen mixed berries.
- Seal and refrigerate overnight. Best used within 2 days.

Tropical Delight Oatmeal Jar:

- Put 1/4 cup steel-cut organic oats* in a wide-mouth mason jar.
- Pour in 3/4 cup milk.
- Top with 1 Tablespoon dried pumpkin seeds, 1 Tablespoon unsweetened coconut, and chunks of dried or frozen mango.

- Seal and refrigerate overnight. Use in 2-3 days.

*Food companies make steel-cut oats by chopping whole oats into little chunks. Steel-cut oats taste nuttier and feel chewier in the mouth than the more typical oatmeal flakes. They also have a lower glycemic index, which means they provide a slower release of energy and help keep blood sugar on a more even keel. One disadvantage of steel-cut oats is that they take longer to cook: up to five minutes in the microwave or ten to thirty minutes on a stovetop. However, I soak them overnight so they only take two minutes in the microwave cooking.

For a Light Day

*Whip up a hot breakfast with vegetables and fruit**

- Scramble two eggs in a small bowl.
- Season with salt and pepper.
- Heat 1 teaspoon olive or peanut oil in a small skillet.
- Add eggs.
- Grab a handful of pre-washed spinach from a bag in the fridge and drop into the skillet.
- Sprinkle thyme and Parmesan cheese on top. Cook eggs until the white and yolks are set.
- Fold in half to make an omelette.

- Serve with a slice of toast drizzled with honey and cinnamon.
- Garnish with fresh orange slices.

*Take a gratitude break before you eat:

- As you peel the orange, squeeze the skin until you get orange essence on your fingers. Breathe it in.
- What memories stir?
- Sit for a moment, and visualize your last trip or vacation. Say a prayer of gratitude... treasure your pleasant memories.

MY STORY

I begin with confessions: I have never been on a diet. I don't have a bathroom scale in my home. I refuse to count my steps. I drink whole milk, love bacon, and relish a piece of dark chocolate for breakfast almost every morning. I struggle with high blood pressure and, at the moment, take medication to manage it.

In short, I am human, and imperfect. But wait, there's more:

I have little natural athletic ability and haven't starred on a sports team of any kind. By a fluke that surprised everyone, I was selected to be a cheerleader for one year in high school and performed so poorly I suffered the humiliation of not being selected the next year. Yet I love to exercise and have made physical activity a regular part of my life, whether during the season when my children were at home and needed chauffeuring to all kinds of sport and school activities, or when I focused on a corporate sales career with extensive travel, or during the year I managed the affairs and care of my terminally ill father.

Last year I finally gave up drinking Coca-Cola, a beverage I have always adored. For years I disliked drinking water and secretly made fun of hydration-obsessed people who carried water bottles everywhere. Now I drink a half cup of water before I go to bed, a full cup first thing in the morning, and I enjoy my own collection of water bottles!

All this is to say that change is possible. None of us should throw up our hands and accept habits that threaten our health just because that's how we are or it's what we've always done. One small success will lead to another if we change our behaviors in small steps that we solidify and turn into automatic habits.

I majored in food and nutrition in college, completed post-graduate training to become a registered dietitian nutritionist (RDN), and worked in hospitals and nursing homes in five different states. When I went back to school for a master's degree in nutrition, I learned much working alongside top-tier doctors and dietitians.

In my personal life, I've watched people I love die from dementia, cancer, kidney disease, and stroke. As I saw the end of life up close, it impressed me that much of what we do in life depends on basic functions we take for granted until we lose them. Goal-oriented professional people like you and me have business plans, financial plans, and life plans. We often spend little time planning for the health of our whole person.

To soar into a productive and successful life you need more than a good HDL cholesterol number and an annual flu vaccine, though both may be important.

Living well depends on the sense of purpose you find in your work, how well you deal with frustration and conflict, how much you sleep, and how you nourish and move your body. It certainly depends on the richness of your friendships.

I wrote this book because I want my friends and readers to live full, joyful lives. Don't survive...thrive!

Accept yourself as you are, but love yourself enough to not want to stay that way. Your life matters, and you need vigorous health so you can burst forth with all the gifts and creations that are your unique offering to the world: the contribution that only you can make.

Key Take Aways and Actions Steps

What action step will you choose? It can be a small step. For example:

- Place a favorite cup or mug by your kitchen sink as a visual cue to drink eight ounces of cold water the first thing every morning.
- Set your alarm fifteen minutes earlier to create time for breakfast.
- Go through your pantry and throw out sugary cereals and sweet pastries.
- Place a grocery order that includes organic steel cut oats, unsalted nuts, and wild frozen blueberries.

Select your next step, and take action today!

Sleep

WE ARE SUCH STUFF AS DREAMS ARE MADE ON; AND OUR LITTLE LIFE IS ROUNDED WITH A SLEEP.

—William Shakespeare

You have probably heard or read that getting a good night's sleep is important for your health. Yet if you are like many high-achieving professionals, you might view scrimping on sleep as a clever way to carve out more time for work. Perhaps you feel proud of your ability to get by on less sleep than other people you know.

With constant connection to media through our digital devices, it seems that more of us have trouble falling or staying asleep. About nine million Americans received prescriptions for zolpidem (brand name Ambien) in 2011.

Poet Wendell Berry wrote in "The Wild Geese" that sleep means "abandon." When we sleep, we must leave our tweets, pins, spreadsheets, and to-do lists, abandon them and slip to a place of no awareness. Is that why we have trouble sleeping? Are we afraid to disconnect? Do we fear missing out?

The Centers for Disease Control says "short sleepers" (those who sleep less than seven hours a night) are more likely to be obese, physically inactive, smoke, and prone to a sobering list of health problems:

- Heart attack
- Cardiovascular disease
- Stroke
- Asthma
- Chronic obstructive pulmonary disease (COPD)
- Cancer
- Arthritis
- Depression
- Chronic kidney disease
- Diabetes

Sleep influences health because our hormone levels and metabolic processes change in response to sleep deprivation. Weight gain, high blood pressure, and diabetes may develop due to these metabolic changes.

For example, when a person does not get enough sleep, levels of ghrelin, a hormone that stimulates hunger, tend to go up, and levels of leptin, a hormone associated with feeling full, go down. Greater hunger because of sleep deprivation could mean you eat more and gain weight. A 2020 study found that women with poor sleep quality consumed more food and calories and had lower diet quality, while a 2018 intervention study indicated sleeping longer resulted in eating less free sugars.

During sleep, blood pressure goes down. With less sleep, the average daily blood pressure remains higher, increasing the risk of heart attack, stroke, and chronic kidney disease.

Even one night of disturbed sleep, such as sleeping less than four hours, has been found to increase production of sugar by the liver and reduce the uptake of blood sugar by other body tissues. Therefore, people deprived of sleep experience higher blood sugar levels, and become more prone to developing type 2 diabetes or experiencing poor blood sugar control if they already have the disease.

Sleep also figures in two other conditions that pose massive future health concerns for Americans and the U.S. health care systems: childhood obesity and Alzheimer's disease.

Health care professionals worry that the percentage of U.S. children and teenagers who are obese has more than tripled since the 1970s.

> *"Childhood obesity is a serious problem in the United States. The obesity epidemic threatens to shorten life expectancy in the United States and bankrupt the health care system.»*
>
> *—Dr. David Ludwig, professor of nutrition at Harvard School of Public Health*

A 2018 study found that children with a regular bedtime routine who got the recommended amount of sleep were more likely to have a healthy body weight when they were teenagers. Sufficient sleep for children was defined as at least eleven hours a night for five year olds, and at least ten hours a night for nine year olds. Those without a consistent bedtime routine at age nine gained 38% more in body mass by age fifteen than those who met the sleep guidelines. For a serious public health concern like obesity, isn't it amazing that something simple like regular bedtime and enough sleep can make a difference?

During sleep, the brain processes the experiences of the day and clears away metabolic toxins that may have accumulated. Adequate sleep improves learning and memory retention. Some researchers associate chronic sleep deprivation with greater risk of neurological disorders like Alzheimer's disease and Parkinson's.

Arranging your life to get enough sleep can give you huge dividends of vigor, calm, and a brighter outlook on life. How are your sleep habits? How much is enough for you? While individual sleep needs vary, most adults need seven to nine hours a night.

If you feel you don't sleep enough, assess if it is because you don't set aside enough time for sleep, or because you struggle to fall or stay asleep. If the first, you may need to re-order your priorities and time commitments. If the second, commit to an evening routine that promotes sleep. Don't wait until it's 11:00p.m. after binge-watching hours of a TV crime show. Plan ahead and set an environment conducive to sleep using ideas from the **Make It Happen** section that follows. Your goal is to make a restful, full night's sleep the automatic, easy choice. With a consistent sleep schedule, you can wake up calm and energetic, ready to win at life like Tom Brady:

> *Proper sleep has helped me get to where I am today as an athlete, and it is something that I continue to rely on every day.*
>
> *— Tom Brady, NFL quarterback and five-time Super Bowl champion*

Many people think that improving your health requires drastic, painful changes such as a sharp curtailment of your food intake, following a special diet that requires the elimination of large groups of foods, or spending a great deal of money on special ingredients and supplements. Isn't it great news that getting more sleep is a powerful, effective way to improve your health?

Evidence about Sleep

1. Zuraikat, F.M., Makarem, N., Liao, M., St.-Onge, M., Aggarwal, B. Measures of Poor Sleep Quality Are Associated With Higher Energy Intake and Poor Diet Quality in a Diverse Sample of Women From the Go Red for Women Strategically Focused Research Network. J Am Heart Assoc. 2020; 9:e014587.
2. Al Khatibi, H.K., Hall, W.L., Creedon, A. Ooi, E., Masri, T., McGowan, L., Harding, S.V.,

Darzi, J., Pot, G.K. Sleep Extension Is a Feasible Lifestyle Intervention in Freeliving Adults Who Are Habitually Short Sleepers: A Potential Strategy for Decreasing Intake of Free Sugars? A Randomized Controlled Pilot Study. Am J Clin Nutr. 2018; 107:43-53.

3. Huang, T., and Redline, S. Cross-sectional and Prospective Associations of Actigraphy-Assessed Sleep Regularity With Metabolic Abnormalities: The Multi-Ethnic Study of Atherosclerosis. Diabetes Care. 2019; 8:1422-1429.
4. Donga, E., van Dijk, M., van Dijk, J.G., Bierfass, N.R., Lammers, G.J., van Kralingen, K.W., Corssmit, E.P.M., Romjin, J.A. A Single Night of Partial Sleep Deprivation Induces Insulin Resistance in Multiple Metabolic Pathways in Healthy Subjects. J Clin Endocrinol Metab. 2010; 95:2963-2968.
5. Lee, S., Hale, L., Chang, A., Nahmod, N.G., Master, L., Berger, L.M., Buxton, O.M. Longitudinal Associations of Childhood Bedtime and Sleep Routines With Adolescent Body Mass Index. Sleep. 2018:1-9.

MAKE IT HAPPEN

How Not to Sleep Like a Baby

We all admire sleeping babies because they appear so serene and sweet. But do you really want to wake up crying every three hours during the night? I didn't think so.

A few years ago, I went to a bicycling event where I slept in a college dorm with other people. After the first night a friend gave me an unusual compliment: "You're a good sleeper." Because there are dire warnings about the consequences of sleep deprivation, I appreciated the compliment.

I want to be gentle with sleep advice, knowing some struggle with insomnia due to factors I may not understand or experience. Perhaps I inherited good sleep patterns from my parents. Both were superb sleepers. Dad could drink black coffee at nine p.m. and fall asleep at ten. Mom slept through family car trips of any length—from five hours to grandma's or four days cross country.

When at home she slept at least nine hours every day, and took a ritual afternoon nap.

Yet even so, at times I toss and turn. These practices help me not sleep like a baby:

S = shut down screens well before bedtime
L = Let go of anger
E = Eliminate stimulants
E = Exercise
P = Prepare for sleep

Shut down screens well before bedtime. The blue light from TVs, computers, and smart phones may stimulate our brains to wakefulness. Do you have a TV in your bedroom, work on email at night, and text until the lights go off? That must stop. To make it an automatic habit, install a timer or sleep controller on your devices. I use the bedtime feature on my IPhone. It plays a bar of Brahms' lullaby and turns off sounds and notifications on my phone at the time I select for bedtime. After that, I don't hear calls or texts, and the screen is dark, so I'm less tempted to surf the internet. If you have a TV in your bedroom, set it to shut down at bedtime, or better yet, move it from your bedroom.

Let go of anger. The Bible says "In your anger do not sin; when you are on your beds, search your hearts and be silent" (Psalms 4:4). How many times do you hash over a situation or carry on an imaginary conversation at night because of unresolved anger or frustration? The psalmist says to be at peace, with a silent heart. That may require courageous and vulnerable conversations, setting and enforcing boundaries, or choosing to love and forgive. Make those choices early in the day. I sleep better if I tackle tough conversations or situations in the morning. If you have trouble sleeping, consider if problems you avoid all day rise up to disturb you at night.

I've also learned that after a certain hour it's best not to accept phone calls that might upset me. That seems quite obvious, but it may be a big change to put into practice. I had to pay a therapist to learn how to do that. In the tough days when my former husband and I were separated, doing our best to fix a fractured marriage, I complained to her that he sabotaged my self-care.

"After work I'll exercise, eat a good dinner, and relax listening to music. As evening approaches I feel good, ready to fall asleep. Then he'll call me around 9:30 p.m. and say he needs to talk about something. Next thing I know, I'm angry and uptight and can't fall asleep for hours," I whined.

She looked at me. "Don't answer the phone if he calls after a certain hour. Tell him if he wishes to talk to you, he needs to call before 7:00 p.m., or whatever time you choose."

Wow. I was so used to responding to everyone's every demand. This was a novel idea.

It worked.

Eliminate stimulants in the evening if you are sensitive to caffeine. Unlike my dad, I respond to minuscule amounts of caffeine and have trouble sleeping if I eat dark chocolate or drink coffee or tea in the evening. Alcohol makes me drowsy, but I don't sleep well after drinking a lot of it because my sleep is restless. If I consume more than one alcoholic beverage, I wake up several times during the night. If your top priority is better sleep, eliminate coffee, tea, caffeinated colas, and booze from your daily routine. Cleanse your pantry by pouring sources of caffeine and alcohol down the drain.

"That sounds drastic!"

Yes. The only way to change your life is to change your habits. The easiest way to change a bad habit is to make it hard to do. If you don't have caffeine or alcohol in the house, you won't consume it in the evening. If you need coffee or tea to come alive in the morning, you can grab a cup from the office break room, stop at a market on the way to work, or order a cup for pickup from a local coffee shop, and enjoy a morning walk to go get it. After you get rid of the shallow sleep that comes from alcohol consumption, you might need less caffeine to jolt yourself awake each morning.

Exercise. This reduces stress and generates whole body calmness. I love the way I feel after exercise. It is sad when healthcare professionals recommend sleep medications more often than they prescribe physical activity for relaxation and restfulness. We'll go deeper into exercise recommendations in a later chapter, but walking, hiking, yoga, and bicycling all drain tension from my body and give me a night of deep, restful sleep.

Prepare for sleep. I wonder how much insomnia in our culture comes from the fast pace at which we live. Often we focus more on DOING than BEING. Going to sleep requires letting go, as Wendell Berry says in his poem "The Wild Geese." Do you have trouble letting go? Do you always push yourself to do more, achieve more, earn more? If so, there are probably evenings you fall into bed with physical exhaustion, yet find you can't go to sleep because your head spins as you think about all the things you need to do. Here are practices that will help you transition from driving ambition to sleepy abandonment:

- Recite and reflect on things for which you're thankful.
- Take ten deep breaths. The yoga practice of ujjayi breath, sometimes called "Darth Vader breath," is explained in the Helpful Tools section at the back of this book. Deep breathing helps your body shift from a stress-driven fight-or-flight response to a slow and rhythmic control of breath and heartbeat.
- Read calming fiction or poetry. At bedtime I like to read books by novelists like Marilynne Robinson, any Wendell Berry novels or poems, or poetry by my friend Sandy Coomer, an essayist in a later chapter of this book. These authors write with beauty and depth, and build scenes I can

imagine with my senses. They create characters that feel like old friends who will always be there for me the next time I pick up the book. I'm entranced, but not driven to an adrenaline high of fear or excitement. Although I also read thrillers and suspenseful dramas, I save them for the weekend, so I'm not revved up and still turning pages at midnight.

- Dab lavender or cedar wood essential oil on your temples, wrists, and the soles of your feet.

And now, here are specific actions to help you sleep better after different types of days.

For a Slammed Day

Turn off your screens—TV, computer, phone—as soon as you can. (If you have a TV in your bedroom, move it TOMORROW.) Adjust your thermostat so your bedroom is about three degrees cooler.

Breathe in, breathe out, stretch. Reach your arms high above your head, and sway from side to side like a palm tree (if that doesn't hurt your back or shoulders).

If you can use and tolerate essential oils, dab lavender or cedar wood oil on each wrist. Sniff.

Repeat a prayer, mantra, or encouraging phrase to yourself. If you live with someone, tell them you love them. If you don't feel loving at the moment, think back to a time when you did, and tell them about a good memory you shared.

If you live alone, think about a good thing that happened today. Go to bed, take seven deep breaths, (ujjayi breaths if you can), and fall asleep.

For a Typical Day

Turn off all screens—TV, computer, phone—thirty minutes before the time you set for sleep.

Put your phone on mute if possible. (I know if you have teenagers who are out you must keep it on to receive their calls.)

Turn the temperature on the thermostat down three degrees. Sit in a comfortable rocking chair, garden chair, or swing on the front porch.

Drink a cup of chamomile tea or room temperature water. Listen to beautiful music or the outdoor sounds of evening. If you live with someone, talk about something good that happened during your day.

If you live alone, recite your wins, accomplishments, and blessings.

Get in bed, do twelve deep breaths (ujjayi breaths if you can), and fall asleep.

For a Light Day

Two hours before bedtime, fix a warm bath, drop in lavender essential oil, select calming music and settle in! (Some experts say a bath immediately before bedtime may make you feel more alert.) A warm bath will increase the time you spend in slow-wave sleep, the deepest, most restorative stage of sleep.

During slow-wave sleep, your brain clears out oxygen byproducts that can damage brain cells. Slow-wave sleep also increases the release of a hormone that promotes growth and repair and supports memory consolidation.

As an example of a beautiful, soothing piece of literature to read at bedtime, here is Wendell Berry's poem "*The Wild Geese*":

Horseback on Sunday morning,
harvest over, we taste persimmon
and wild grape, sharp sweet
of summer's end. In time's maze
over fall fields, we name names
that went west from here, names
that rest on graves. We open
a persimmon seed to find the tree
that stands in promise,
pale, in the seed's marrow.
Geese appear high over us,
pass, and the sky closes. Abandon,
as in love or sleep, holds
them to their way, clear,
in the ancient faith: what we need
is here. And we pray, not
for new earth or heaven, but to be
quiet in heart, and in eye
clear. What we need is here.

May you end each day with quiet heart and clear eye, and abandon yourself to a deep, restorative sleep.

STEPHANIE'S STORY

I began to struggle with insomnia after the birth of my first child. I became so used to being forced awake that when my baby started sleeping through the night (and I mean, eleven hours straight at six months!) I would still wake between two and four in the morning. The fact that he was sleeping and I could not was head-wrecking. I began obsessive night checking to make sure he had not stopped breathing from SIDS, or been abducted in his sleep like a kiddie pageant queen. I would lie awake imagining all the things that could happen... or wondering how he would turn out, or whether or not we were making the right decisions about the myriad hot button parenting issues that loom large in the mind of a first-time mother.

Worry became my constant companion, and this only intensified after the birth of my second child, who had multiple disabilities. When he was three, he developed epilepsy, and that started another, this time very concrete, set of concerns. I began creeping into his room to make sure he wasn't seizing.

Fragmented sleep had been the norm for many years. Every night I would wake between two and four o'clock. Every night I would be up for hours, usually nodding off right before my early risers summoned me to start the day. My husband traveled for work almost constantly, which piled even more on my sagging plate.

The problem with insomnia is that it begets insomnia. The more you can't sleep, the more you worry about not being able to sleep. Perversely, sleep deprivation makes winding down even harder to do. I begged God to let me sleep. I asked friends to pray for me, then they would ask how I was sleeping, which then made me more anxious about not sleeping. I scoured the internet for solutions, trying vitamins, yoga, herbs, amber-colored glasses, and other non-pharmaceutical hacks to try to sleep through the night. Nothing worked, and the harder I tried, the worse it got. Being an insomniac became part of my identity.

It was then that I realized my problem... it was the trying. I needed to stop the trying. The research, the hacks, the talking about it. All the things that had made me successful in school—research! Reading! Trying! REALLY hard!

These things were not serving me in the sleep department. I began to surrender to my insomnia. I decided not to worry about it anymore. I stopped talking about it. I stopped the nightly rounds to check on the kids or make sure the doors were locked and the lights turned off. I just let being awake in the night be an okay thing. I trusted that God would give me the sleep I needed for whatever was on tap for the following day. I reminded myself that I would get through the day, and I did, and I do.

The shift didn't happen right away, but now, most nights, I sleep. My son still has epilepsy. My husband still travels. My circumstances haven't changed particularly, but I changed. I let go, and in doing so, I found what I needed.

—Stephanie Hsiang has degrees from Smith College and The University of Edinburgh. She is a wife and a stay-at-home mom of two boys, one dog, eight chickens, and countless probiotic pets. She is also an exercise enthusiast, student of interior design, and recovering overachiever. Her greatest achievement on any given day is keeping everyone alive.

Key Take Aways and Action Steps

What is your next action step toward better sleep?

Journal

KEEPING A JOURNAL OF WHAT'S GOING ON IN YOUR LIFE IS A GOOD WAY TO HELP YOU DISTILL WHAT'S IMPORTANT AND WHAT'S NOT.

—Martina Navratilova, former professional tennis player and coach, widely considered one of the best female tennis players of all time

Since you're busy and already have too much to do, why should you spend twenty precious minutes of your day writing to yourself? What can that do for you?

Journaling can change your life, your health, and your personal and business success. Throughout history, a large number of super achievers praised the habit of journaling every day. Hear what a few of them have to say about journaling:

Starting a gratitude journal was the single most important thing I have ever done.

—Oprah Winfrey, talk show host, actress, television producer, media executive, and philanthropist

If you're serious about becoming a wealthy, powerful, sophisticated, ***healthy,*** *influential, cultured, and unique individual, keep a journal. (Emphasis mine.)*

—Jim Rohn, the late entrepreneur, author, and speaker who rose from a childhood of poverty as a farm boy and college dropout to mentor Tony Robbins and Jack Canfield, and amass a net worth of $500 million

What happens to us is not as important as the meaning we assign to it. Journaling helps sort this out.

—Michael Hyatt, CEO, entrepreneur, author of a New York Times best seller and two Wall Street Journal best sellers

I can shake off everything as I write; my sorrows, disappear, my courage is reborn.

—Anne Frank, a fifteen-year-old named one of Time Magazine's 100 Most Important People of the Century

To consider what journaling may do for you, ask yourself these questions:

- How well do I understand my feelings?
- What circumstances make me feel confused and bewildered?
- Are there people I want to confront, but I don't know what to say?

- Do I have a decision to make, and I can't figure out what to do?
- Is there a loss that drags me into despair and depression at unexpected moments?
- Am I scared about something?

Journaling can help you deal with loneliness, confusion, difficult people, tough decisions, loss, and fear. Many famous people journaled—Albert Einstein, Mark Twain, Thomas Edison, and Bridget Jones! Journaling is critical to wellness because it helps you connect to your core, the inner essence that gets drowned out and ignored and covered up by everything else you have to do in life.

You may feel you already have too much to do. How can you find time to journal? You know you're supposed to exercise, and you don't have the willpower. Your schedule is so crazy you don't plan meals or cook much. Surely those things are more important than journaling?

Maybe.

I believe that journaling, day after day, year after year, helps you know yourself. Knowing yourself lets you see how you spend your time. When you see that with clarity, your perspective shifts, and your vision expands so you think of one small change you will make in your habits. After that change you feel calmer, or less worn down, or more hopeful. You embark on a path of growth.

You begin a process that transforms you.

Several years ago I traveled to lush and beautiful Kiawah Island, South Carolina, to escape the deep grief and depression I suffered after my father died and I lost my job. One evening I stood on the beach at dusk as the sun slipped below the horizon and the water turned a choppy steel gray. In front of me, all I could see was the crash and spray of the pounding surf. Then I lifted my gaze and looked further out to sea. Beyond a certain point, the ocean was calm and flat. It was as smooth as a sheet of glass. I gasped, then smiled. I felt Mother Nature had sent me a message. My life was rough and choppy at the moment, but there would be smooth sailing in my future.

Perhaps you've had similar experiences—a time when a trip to a new place gave you a new outlook on life. It may have been when you stood on a massive mountain peak and watched an eagle soar in clear air and heard the wind rustle through tree leaves, or when you shimmied and danced with joy at a concert with your favorite band, or when you smelled the sweet perfume of clean baby skin. Something happened, and *POOF*. You saw things in a different way.

I hope you get to go to the beach or the mountain or the concert or smell the baby and get your *POOF*. Those are incredible, but occasional, experiences.

Journaling is a way to get mountain-top POOFs every day as you spill uncensored thoughts, ideas, and feelings into a notebook. Journaling can change your life and help you build consistent healthy habits. In the essay part of this chapter, I will tell about a time journaling kept me going when I wanted to stop. But next, a few practical tips that make journaling easy and painless.

Evidence about Journaling

1. Mueller, P.A., and Oppenheimer, D.M. The Pen Is Mightier Than the Keyboard: Advantages of Longhand Over Laptop Note Taking. Psychol Sci 2014; 25:1159-1168.
2. Jacobs, R. The Way In: Journal Writing for Self-Discovery. United States: Sharmor Editions, 2010.
3. Environmental Protection Agency. Candles and Incense As Potential Sources of Indoor Air Pollution: Market Analysis And Literature Review. 2001; https://cfpub.epa.gov/
4. Massoudi, R., and Hamidi, A. Emission Products of Petroleum-Based Candles. American Chemical Society National Meeting 2009, Washington D.C. (Abstract).

MAKE IT HAPPEN

Make Journaling a Daily Habit

On the surface, it seems easy to journal ("I'll just grab a notebook and write down a few thoughts when I get a chance"), but the simplicity means it's easy to put off and forget in the press of your many other responsibilities. Pick a specific time of day to journal and commit to it. In my opinion, it's best to journal either last thing at night or first thing in the morning. I like morning because fresh ideas often come to me while I journal and I can put them into practice the same day.

Select journaling tools and use them only for that purpose. I journal with pen and paper because I like the physical act of producing something I can hold, save, and pick up ten or fifteen years later. Scientists say the mind-body connection of writing with pen and paper instead of a computer improves the retention and processing of what we write. When I journal, scribbling whatever comes to my mind without thinking about it ahead of time, quite often a new idea or forgotten detail pops into my awareness. I gain a new perspective.

There are good digital or electronic journals available, but who knows what technology we'll be using in fifteen years? More than once I've flipped through an old journal, either by happenstance as I moved it from one bookshelf to another, or with intent as I tried to find out the day or month something happened. I discovered details I'd forgotten. That may not be possible if an electronic journal sits in an obsolete format. You can also be distracted from the task of journaling if your digital journal lets you see notifications and calls coming to your device. However, a digital journal is more portable and lets you access it any time you have online access. It can be set to give you a reminder. Either method can work, so pick the approach you like best.

If you journal with notebook and pen, buy good quality products you enjoy using. I like the Classic Collection Moleskines with a soft cover. They are durable, but light enough that they don't add much heft to my bag when I travel. I use good roller ball pens from an office supply store.

What do you write when you journal? If you've never journaled and you fear you won't be able to decide what to say, start with a simple format like a gratitude journal. Every day, list three to five things for which you are grateful. Gradually expand to writing details about the things you're grateful for, and why. Try not to write a news report of everything you did the day before. That can feel like work. Journaling is easier and more satisfying when it is a free-flowing stream of thoughts. When you're ready to move past the gratitude journal stage, let your pen fly with whatever comes to mind. Write whatever ideas pour out without conscious planning or preparation. If you're troubled by indecision and weighty decisions you need to make, write about that. Don't force yourself to come up with a solution in your journal. Write about your confusion, your conflicting thoughts, what you want and what you fear. Often you'll gain clarity and insight that will lead you to a decision.

In the end, it doesn't matter how you journal, just that you do. Daily writing helps you notice your thoughts and feelings and observe your reactions to the world around you. As you become more aware, you will begin to glimpse small steps you can take to release stress. You forge habits that produce the energy, calm, and growth that make life more fun and meaningful.

For a Slammed Day

On a crazy busy day, it works best to embed a short journaling activity into something you already do every day. You always take a bath or shower, right?

When you emerge from the bath or shower, wrap yourself in a towel or put on your robe.

If you have a bathroom fan, turn it on to block other noise from the house.

Sit on the toilet seat, grab your journal, and write one page.

That's it. Go forth and conquer your day.

For a Typical Day

After you get up, drink a cup of cold water and fix a mug of coffee or tea.

If others in the house are likely to disturb you, take your mug and journal to a quiet place (front porch, back porch, bedroom, or garage).

If you have infants or young children at home, carve out journaling time by getting up before they do. It will be worth it, for it prepares you to take control of the day. They will control the day if you don't.

Sit in a comfortable position (cross-legged on the floor is good if your back, hips, and knees allow that without pain or discomfort). Place your hands on your knees, close your eyes and take three deep breaths.

In...out

In...out

In...out

If your shoulders are healthy, rotate them up to your ears, back behind you, and around to the front three times.

Up...behind...around Up...behind...around Up... behind...around

Smile.

Then pick up your journal and write.

Stop every now and then and sip your coffee or tea.

For a Light Day

A light day assumes you do not need to hide somewhere to find peace and quiet.

Drink a cup of water and fix yourself a special kind of coffee or tea.

You could grind fresh coffee beans, or brew a special green tea to a specific water temperature and brew time. Use a favorite mug for the coffee, or serve tea in a beautiful china cup.

Sit on a comfy rug before a window, or in your favorite rocking chair on the front porch.

Watch the sun come up, or the dew on the grass.

Are birds singing? Listen to them.

Put before you a plate holding smudged dried herbs, or a cotton ball on which you dripped your favorite essentials oils.*

Sip, sniff, and write a vision of what you want your life to be like in three years. Be specific. Describe what you do, how you live, and with whom you spend your time.

Close your eyes and visualize yourself experiencing the scenes you portrayed. How do you feel?

Focus on that image and feeling for a minute.

See yourself in the scene.

Finish your beverage, sniff the essential oils again, and stretch.

*I used to light a candle and place it in front of me as I journaled. Then I read reports that many candles are made from paraffin wax, which creates toxic chemicals such as benzene and toluene when they burn. These are the same toxins found in diesel fuel fumes. Some people believe the indoor air pollution produced from scented candles is as harmful as second-hand cigarette smoke.

Beeswax candles may be a less polluting alternative for candles, but I use essential oils. The Helpful Tools section has a link to my favorite source for essential oils.

MY STORY

Twenty years ago, my marriage to my college sweetheart ended. I moved from our lovely home into a dusty, mouse-infested farmhouse that sat alone on many acres. It belonged to Elia Kazan, the famed Broadway and Hollywood director and producer. He and his family had used it as a summer home. As the place where Marlon Brando and Vivien Leigh once came for weekend visits and house parties, it held unique charisma and charm. Still, I felt isolated and lonely and sometimes quite scared living there alone.

Even worse was the discovery that I wasn't totally alone. I celebrate holidays by setting out bowls of the special colored M&Ms for each season. One morning I came downstairs to the entry hall and gasped to see that the bowl on my bookcase where I kept red and green Christmas M&Ms was empty. I'd filled the bowl just the previous evening. Who knew mice liked M&Ms, and could eat them so well? If they climbed that high and ate so well, were they rats? I shuddered at the possibilities.

While I lived there, a dear friend gave me Sarah Ban Breathnach's *Simple Abundance A Daybook of Comfort and Joy*. Sarah published this charming book in 1995 to share her journey from frazzled, "workaholic, careaholic perfectionist" to a happy, contented woman who "lived in a state of grace." She wrote a different inspiration for each day of the year. On January 14, I read about a gratitude journal. Sarah said to buy the prettiest, most inviting blank book I could find, and every night before I went to bed to write down five things I was grateful for about my day. She said the gratitude journal was not an option, for I could not transform my life without gratitude.

I started a gratitude journal, and I kept it up. At the time I was depressed. I see that now, but back then I did not realize it. I just felt horrible and unhappy. On many days I did not want to get out of bed to go to my job conducting quality assurance audits in nursing homes around the state. I forced myself to go, but often felt miserable as I drove into the parking lot of each facility.

Then I would start on my rounds. I went into the rooms of paralyzed people who communicated by moving a mouthpiece to point at letters on a computer screen. I saw stroke victims who had to get nutrition through a feeding tube. I visited people with painful, non-healing wounds, and alert, cheerful individuals who greeted me with a smile and shared news of their day. They seemed to be well-adjusted, but as I left the property in my company car I often asked myself: *would they like to have the freedom I have, the opportunity to get in a car and go where they want, when they want?*

On some evenings my gratitude journal looked like this:

I am grateful that:

1. *I can talk*
2. *I can walk*

3. *I can feed myself*
4. *I have a car*
5. *I can drive my car wherever I want to go*

As I wrote in my gratitude journal every day, I began to feel grateful for other things: my children, my friends, the love and support of my parents and siblings, my job, my dog, and many other good things I tended to overlook.

I changed because of gratitude journaling. You can, too. If you want better health, greater fitness, more energy, peace and calm, greater satisfaction with your work, and better relationships with yourself and others—journal.

If it worked for Oprah and it worked for me, it will work for you.

Key Take Aways and Action Steps

Do you journal?

If you do, what do you like most about it?

If you don't, fill in the blanks in the following sentence:

Starting tomorrow, I will use _______to write in a journal at this time __________while I relax in this place __________.

Order

IT IS NOT ENOUGH TO BE BUSY. SO ARE THE ANTS. THE QUESTION IS: WHAT ARE WE BUSY ABOUT?

—Henry David Thoreau

To set yourself up for success in health, happiness, and business, it's important to master two key strategies—time management and organization of your environment. Combined, these describe a life of order.

Time management is a lot about what you decide not to do. Environmental organization means orchestrating the processes of your life so the healthy, stress-reducing actions are the easier, more automatic choices. These components of order reduce the demands and decision fatigue of your day, and help you avoid getting burned out.

The best time management advice I have ever adopted is this: *Every day, cross something off your to-do list and decide not to do it.*

The second-best time management advice, in my opinion, I learned from author and philanthropist Bob Goff in his book *Love Does: Discover a Secretly*

Incredible Life in an Ordinary World. Goff said to make every Thursday quitting day. That means that every Thursday you stop doing something that is not in line with your priorities or is no longer healthy and productive for you.

If you do these two things, improving your health becomes easier. You have more time. Fewer activities compete with your healthy choices.

These ideas illustrate the 80/20 approach to life, a concept derived from a scientific and mathematical model called the Pareto Principle.

Vilfredo Pareto was an Italian philosopher and economist of the late 1800s.

One day he observed that 20% of the pea plants in his garden yielded 80% of the healthy pea pods. Then he discovered that 80% of the land in Italy was owned by 20% of the people. Intrigued, he studied a variety of industries, groups, and phenomena, and found that the 80/20 ratio held true in every one. He concluded:

80% of results come from
just 20% of the actions.

As a young health care professional and medical researcher, I thought time management meant I needed to be efficient and get more done in a given amount of time. So I organized my activities, packed things into a tight schedule, and rushed from one thing to another to make sure I got things done. The problem was, I often didn't enjoy what I did because I felt constant pressure to cross one thing off my to-do list and move on to the next.

Looking back on this period in my life, I saw that I cycled through several stages of work. After weeks or months working at my intense pace, I crashed. Perhaps I got sick and quarantined myself or burned out and morphed from superwoman to a couch-potato-binge-watching-eat-the-whole-carton-of-chocolate-ice-cream slacker. Sometimes I rebelled at the lack of fun in my life. I threw away my to-do list, ditched my goals, and drifted.

Then I learned about the Pareto Principle during a sales leadership course sponsored by my employer. I heard that in the business-to-business sales world, 80% of sales come from 20% of the clients. When I focused my efforts toward that 20%, I succeeded. Later, as a sales manager, I discovered that 80% of the growth in my region would likely come from 20% of my sales people. I used that to guide how I spent my time and who I worked with most often. Year after year, our sales grew.

Now let's consider ways to apply the Pareto Principle to your personal growth and well-being. What would it mean for your lifestyle, finances, and personal life if you honed your focus to the 20% of your actions that produced 80% of the results you sought?

In your business, have you identified your 20% clients? Are you clear about what they need, what they want from you, and how you can improve their customer experience? If you re-orient and prioritize your resources toward the 20% clients, your business will grow.

In your relationships, 80% of your hassles and frustrations come from 20% of your friends. Eighty percent of your joy and encouragement comes from another 20% of your friends. Different people populate these two groups. Spend less time with the first group, and more time with the second. You will enjoy life more and feel less stress.

In your kitchen, it's likely that 80% of your high-calorie/low-nutrient food intake comes from 20% of the foods. Get them out! Throw or give them away. Don't buy them again. For me, salty snacks, like Ruffles potato chips and French onion dip, Cheetos, or caramel corn, always lead me to eat more than I want. As a result, I don't let these foods in my house. There are still times when I crave them, usually late at night while watching a movie. At those times I may regret my disciplined shopping practices, but under the approach known as intentional eating I don't prohibit myself from eating any food. I know that if I want something, I can always have it. However, since I don't routinely keep those foods in the house, there are not many nights I want them enough to leave the sofa, don presentable clothes, get in my car, and drive to the market. It does happen every now and then, especially since I moved to a neighborhood within walking distance of a gas station and market. One Saturday night around 8:30 p.m., as many people bought beer or cigarettes for their weekend, I walked in and plunked a single-serve packet of Ruffles potatoes chips on the counter.

"That will be $1.09," said the clerk. Then, "Is that all you're buying?" "Yes," I said. "Since you don't carry French onion dip."

(I came up with a good imitation of the dip at home by combining unflavored yogurt, finely diced red onions, garlic powder, Parmesan cheese, and Worcestershire sauce.)

In regards to exercise, what 20% of your workouts gives you the most joy AND the greatest boost in cardiovascular fitness and strength? I have seen friends embark on ambitious, extremely challenging exercise programs they end up hating, can't keep up because it's not practical for their schedule, or abandon when they get sidelined with an injury. In contrast, pleasant walks with the dog after work help you decompress after a stressful day and may be easier to maintain. Once you've established a certain baseline of fitness, adding three one-minute intervals of running to a thirty-minute walk can accelerate the cardiovascular and neurological benefits of fitness without adding much time to your workout. Finding a fitness buddy to work out with is another approach that creates a double boost of fitness and stronger connection with a friend.

If you believe you don't have enough time to exercise, or not enough "willpower" to stick with a healthy eating plan, the Pareto Principle helps you identify time-consuming commitments that drain your energy but don't give much back. Quitting something every

Thursday reminds you there are only twenty-four hours in a day. If every time you add a new activity you choose another to let go, you will find it much easier to make time for healthy, stress-draining habits.

In addition to following the Pareto Principle, take a look at your environment and consider what factors influence you so the healthy choice is the easiest choice. Let's consider a simple example.

Imagine I came home from work hungry and tired after a long stressful day and saw a beautiful cake with elegant frosting on the kitchen counter. It was left over from my son's birthday celebration the prior weekend. I cut a generous slice, fixed myself a glass of milk or an adult beverage, and ate cake. Afterward, I remembered my goal to eat less sugar, and wished I had not eaten the cake. "I just have no willpower," I said to myself with disappointment. My spouse was working late that night, so I decided to go ahead and eat dinner. I opened the fridge, but it was bare, holding only a six-pack of beer, wilted lettuce, a carton of eggs, and a package of moldy cheese. I called my hubby. "Hey babe! Coming home soon? Great. There's not much to eat here. How about you stop and pick something up? Sure, BBQ. Yes, onion rings, too. Umm, get me the key lime pie." In this scenario, my hunger combined with the cake on display made eating cake the easiest choice. Then I felt like I'd failed my goal. With no other good options before me, I went all in on the dinner order.

What if my environment had led me in a different direction? For my son's birthday, I bought cupcakes from the best bakery in town, one cupcake for each person attending his party. I enjoyed the cupcake I ate at this special event!

There was nothing left over. I left work feeling hungry after a long, stressful day, but I stopped at the recreation center where I have a membership and changed into the workout clothes I placed in my car that morning. I filled the water bottle in my workout bag with cold, fresh water from the dispensers at the center, enjoyed a vigorous work out, then sat on the floor stretching while I drank more water and talked to friends who also work out there. When I got home I grabbed an apple from the gorgeous bowl of fruit on the kitchen counter— apples, oranges, and pears are there for me to choose—and snacked on the apple and a handful of almonds while I checked in with my spouse. He worked late but was about to head home so I decided I had time to fix something for us both. I looked at the list of four twenty-minute meals stuck to the refrigerator door. I knew all the ingredients were available because I'd placed a set order with the grocery that delivers every Monday. I picked a meal and started on dinner.

When my spouse walked in, it was almost ready. By the time he changed out of his work clothes, dinner was done. We carried it outside and ate on the patio. It was a calm, peaceful meal.

This meal was possible because I set up my environment to make it the easier path. I crossed "go to the grocery" off my to-do list because I have a grocery list in my phone that I order with the touch of a key. I exercised in the time I saved by not going to the grocery, and I didn't get sidetracked by impulse purchases as I trekked all the way to the back of the store to buy a carton of milk for my morning coffee. (All stores put milk in the farthest back corner so shoppers have to walk by everything else to get there.)

The reality is, you don't need time management or willpower if you orient your environment so the healthy options are easy choices. Pick one thing you will change, and redesign your environment so it supports your goal. Make the new behavior automatic. Do it every day, or every week. Soon it requires no decision or thought from you. It is just the way you do things. Since you do it on autopilot, it doesn't require willpower.

Then pick another thing to redesign.

Evidence about Order:

1. Goff, B. Love Does: Discover a Secretly Incredible Life in an Ordinary World. Nashville: Thomas Nelson; 2012.
2. Chu, M. Why Your Environment is the Biggest Factor in Changing Your Life. https://www.inc.com/melissa-chu/its-possible-to-design-your-environment-to-help-yo.html

MAKE IT HAPPEN

Use the 80/20 Rule to Create Order in Your Life

How do you know which 20% of your choices and actions give you the most reward? Our lives are fluid, complex, and intangible. They can't be measured as easily as an accountant reconciles the books, or a factory manager tallies production. You'll have to do some detective-like sleuthing in your life. You can do this in one of two ways: look ahead at your schedule, or record your reaction to your activities as you live them. We'll discuss the look-ahead method first and modify a method made famous by Marie Kondo, author of *The Life-Changing Magic of Tidying Up: The Japanese Art of Decluttering and Organizing.*

Find a quiet place where you can sit for about twenty minutes without interruption. Look at your calendar for the next week and make a list of all activities outside of work or exercise. Rate each either 1, 2,or 3.

1 = Wow. To quote Marie, this sparks joy.

2 = OK. Not exciting, but part of my routine.

3 = Ugh. If I could do something else I would.

Do this for four weeks in a row until you have a list that represents how you spend your time. If you want a quicker start, look back at your calendar for the past month and go through the same procedure. Write down the number threes in a new list and look them over. Which ones may be difficult or tiring but align with your core values? Cross these off the list and put them aside for now. You may need to find a way to share the responsibility or get help bearing up, but many difficult activities do spark joy in the end because they give deep meaning and value.

During the nine months my father was dying of cancer, I dreaded each solo 230-mile drive from my home to his. I didn't like assuming management of his affairs or taking calls from his physicians or hospice nurses. Now, I am grateful for every moment I spent with him in his last months. I was healed by the conversations we shared, by our sly jokes and sweet hugs. If you can, don't quit a difficult activity that serves a core value. Revise your approach, ask for help, find an easier way, but don't quit.

Next, pick up your journal and skim through the pages. You are journaling, aren't you? If you aren't, return to Chapter 3 for a primer on the benefits of journaling. Look for reoccurring rants. Which friend seems to set off conflict or drama over and over? Does your softball team or your PTA or the colleague with whom you work often make the news in your journal? Add to your number three list any repeated mentions from your journal EXCEPT immediate family members. Of course you want your spouse, parents, siblings, and children to be among the 20% who reward and delight you. I hope they do, but life can be difficult, and that is not always the case. Consider seeking professional help to work through troubled family bonds, and seek healing for yourself from deep hurts or trauma in your past that still loom in your present interactions with others. Many people can benefit from counseling at some point; however, I am not equipped to address psychological or emotional issues from relationships, nor provide therapy or counseling.

I have found it necessary to step away from people I've known and loved for years, often after a challenging time in life transforms my perspective and priorities and makes me notice things I had not seen before. This type of quitting is hard and painful. The Bible describes how our focus changes as we grow:

> *When I was a child, I talked like a child, I thought like a child, I reasoned like a child. When I became a man, I put childish ways behind me.*
>
> *—I Corinthians 13:11*

When I was more insecure and in need of acceptance from others, I often adapted myself to gain the approval of bright and shiny "stars." I gravitated toward them as friends. As I got stronger and learned to like myself more, I changed. I spoke up for what I wanted. I desired to be heard and to live my own life instead of orienting so much around my friends' stories and dramas. I noticed details about how some people treated me. In a few instances, I saw that stories we'd laughed about for years were disrespectful, neglectful, or on occasion, emotionally abusive. I found that as I grew, not everyone around me wanted to adjust to the changes that ensued. If you find people in your journal who set you off on a regular basis, and you have tried to reach understanding with them but couldn't, you may need to put them on your number three list.

Now, make Thursday your "quitting day."

If you keep a to-do list, look at the items you vowed to do at the start of the week. If it's not done by Thursday, ask yourself:

"Does it need to be done? How much growth and progress comes from this?"

Go down your to-do list and pick an item you determine doesn't need to be done or doesn't produce much positive result. Cross it off the list or delegate it to someone else.

Now look at the number three list you made after reviewing your calendar and journal. Which activity or contact gives you the least joy, fails to satisfy a deep value, or creates the most frustration and tension? Pick the clearest choice and consider ways to let it go.

If it's a co-worker, is it possible to change your schedule so you don't cross paths as often, move to a new office setting, work from home, or (in severe cases) transfer to another position? One caveat: don't get in the habit of moving because of difficult people. Some of the hardest work situations I've face helped me learn valuable skills and lessons and improved my career progression for years afterward. Make sure you've approached the situation asking what you can learn, how you could adopt a different approach, what does this person have to teach you? As Stephen Covey wrote in his book *The 7 Habits of Highly Effective People*,

> *Seek first to understand,*
> *then to be understood.*

There may be someone just like this person in your next job! Yet, if you've tried everything you can without success, and the work situation causes you to lose sleep, be moody and unhappy with your family and friends, beware. Chronic stress wreaks havoc on our bodies. It increases blood pressure, which can lead to heart or kidney disease, and increases blood sugar and insulin resistance, which leads to diabetes. Chronic stress contributes to weight and fat gain from high cortisol levels and suppresses immunity which makes you more susceptible to infections or even cancer. A healthy habit may involve leaving a toxic situation.

If your most obvious number three is an ongoing commitment, such as a volunteer position, community committee, club or sporting activity, it can be easy to quit once you see the need. There are many activities we continue doing for no reason other than we've done them for years. We don't stop to evaluate if they are the best use of our time now, in the present.

I played recreational tennis for years. I joined teams, drilled and practiced every week at set times, and went to tennis camps with friends. My children learned not to disturb Mom when a grand-slam professional tennis tournament was on TV! Each time we relocated, I found a tennis league right away and through that met people and made friends. I was a stay-at-home mom when I started tennis, but I kept it up with a standing Tuesday morning court time after I returned to work part-time. When I took a full-time job in medical sales, Tuesday morning tennis at 9:30 stayed in my schedule for seven years (the beauty of remote work!)

As my career progressed and I moved into more demanding jobs and relocated twice more, I switched to tennis at night but kept trying to play. I would rush home from a work trip to throw on my tennis clothes and barrel down the road to get to a match on time. I didn't get to know the other women on my team. We played, then went our separate ways.

One day, I realized tennis was no longer a source of joy for me. It had become a source of stress, one more demand on a long to-do list. When I began tennis, the intricacy of doubles and the competitive thrill of smashing a forehand down the line exercised my strategic thinking and satisfied an urge to compete that was missing from my life as a stay-at-home mom. Now, I developed strategies for million-dollar customers and fought to win deals. I needed hobbies that brought peace and relaxation, rather than competition and stimulation. The sport I loved no longer worked for me.

I quit tennis and took up more serene pursuits like yoga, bicycling, and flat-water kayaking. It was an excellent decision and I have felt much happier ever since.

When we set intentions or goals, we are adding new things we want to do.

We want to learn this, or become more that, or take on such-and-such project. As we add, we must also let go. Otherwise, our purpose in life and our deepest desires and intentions get lost in a flurry of busyness. Life becomes a list of obligations to endure. We dream about things we'd like to do "someday," but we don't get around to doing them because we are so busy.

My friend: someday is now. It is OK to make changes. Let go.

Quit.

Breathe.

Take a walk, and notice where you are.

When in doubt, recite this quote from Steve Jobs:

> *People think focus means saying yes to the things you've got to focus on. But that's not what it means at all. It means saying no to the hundred other good ideas that there are. You have to pick carefully. I'm actually as proud of the things we haven't done as the things I have done. Innovation means saying no to 1,000 things.*

AMY'S STORY

In February 2014, I decided to put my lengthy experience in nonprofit to use in the for-profit world. Having developed a unique skill set, including living and working in Africa, I wanted to practice international development in a different way. Taking my passion for tourism, combined with my human rights work and my deep commitment to wildlife conservation, I started my own business. I founded Flyga Twiga™ a personal safari service, focusing on Southern and East Africa.

Having worked from home before, most of the first year went smoothly. With all the excitement that comes from a new venture, it was easy to manage my time well. Then in November, I received a text from my husband. The text read, "How would you like to go to South Korea?" I immediately said "yes." By December 31st I was on a Korean Air flight to South Korea.

The first few months of 2015 were a whirlwind of our soaking up every experience our new home had to offer. Schedules for my business went out the window.

But, as the whirlwind "our new home" honeymoon phase wound down, it was then I was hit by how out of control my time management for my business had become. Spending days at home, without the support network I had had in the States, meant drifting from one thought to the next, without order. In addition, in South Korea I was 12-13 hours ahead of the network I had come to rely upon.

It was time to realign my priorities. But how? This was my first experience as an entrepreneur, working from home alone. I was the boss to whom I must answer. I had one tool in my toolbox which had never failed me, walking.

Walking is what I did.

Following the Korean War, Seoul quickly rebuilt. The powerful South Korean workforce put all its energy into building what was to become one of the most robust economies on earth. By the early 1980s Seoul had matured to the point of self-reflection. What did it mean to live in a healthy urban environment? One answer was the creation of Hangang Park. A series of 12 parks, Hangang Park encourages the citizens of Seoul to be outdoors and lead a healthy lifestyle. In addition to exercise equipment sprinkled throughout the parks, there are a perfectly maintained series of biking and walking paths.

With Hangang Park at my doorsteps, to relieve the stress and put some structure back into my life, I began each day walking. I added to this listening to uplifting motivational podcasts, often focusing on business growth. Within a week, my commitment to walking began to even out my time management. By clearing my head and calmly beginning the day, structure flowed through the rest of the day. And, indeed, I found a benefit many business owners find from walking: my creative juices began flowing.

By making a morning walk my top priority, I was able to focus clearly on the working hours ahead in my home office. Structure and order began the day.

Time management through physical movement is definitely an awesome way to improve your business and your quality of life!

—Flyga Twiga™ is a Personal Safari Service founded in 2014 by Amy Millican. Amy helps you plan your perfect African Safari! Having lived and worked throughout East and Southern Africa, including with Wildlife Conservation Society - South Sudan, Amy helps you create your dream, bespoke African Safari. Your adventure starts here: www.flygatwiga.com

Key Take Aways and Action Steps

What relationships, activities, and commitments add stress but generate very little joy?

What action will you take to change your approach toward them? What will you give up this Thursday?

Nature

EVEN FIVE MINUTES AROUND TREES OR IN GREEN SPACES MAY IMPROVE HEALTH. THINK OF IT AS A PRESCRIPTION WITH NO SIDE EFFECTS THAT'S ALSO FREE.

—New York State Department of Environmental Conservatism

It was a cold, windy Sunday afternoon in March when I walked Manhattan's High Line for the first time. Even though it was not a pretty day, the path was packed! Hundreds of people ambled along the concrete surface converted to an urban walkway. Constructed in 1934 as an elevated railway to get vehicles carrying food into lower Manhattan off the streets, by the 1990s the High Line was an abandoned eyesore littered with trash and an overgrown tangle of wild plants.

I adored the High Line and the chance to see open sky, admired the trees, ornamental grasses and flowerbeds that now decorate its path, and relished escaping the noise and congestion of city streets below. Even so, it seemed a paltry piece of nature on which to walk, compared to the Sierra Mountains of California, the spacious beauty of the desert Southwest, or the forests and fields surrounding my home in Tennessee. When I saw how many New Yorkers risked cold and discomfort to be outside that afternoon, I realized we humans must hunger for contact with the natural world, even as modern life becomes more automated and artificial. Current research suggests spending time in natural surroundings not only feels good, but is good for us. "Nature bathing," to paraphrase the Japanese expression "shinrin-yoku," is trendy because being in nature enhances our health.

Isn't that amazing?

We live in an era when scans see inside your organs, health care professionals hundreds of miles away can track your breathing and heart rate, and you can wave a device over your arm to check your blood sugar without drawing a drop of blood. With such advances in technology, can something as simple as a walk in a forest can improve your health?

Yes, it can.

Scientists from Japan, Finland, and Korea explain that our bodies are natural, physical entities, and theorize that living in an artificial urban environment creates a state of constant high stress. Returning to nature restores the body. It sounds far-fetched (isn't it enough to enjoy fresh air and sunshine and peace and quiet without expecting miracle health benefits?) but scientific papers document impressive objective findings.

For example, middle-aged employees taken on a three-day, two-night forest trip had a 56% increase in natural killer cell activity, which is a type of white blood cell. They maintained a level 23% higher than baseline even after 23 days back in urban life. Natural killer cells destroy tumor- or virus-infected cells.

Scientists conclude that excursions to the forest seem to fortify immune function.

Our bodies produce a hormone called cortisol when stressed. In times of danger, increased cortisol gives us strength and energy to fight or flee. However, when cortisol levels are high all the time (as happens with chronic stress), we gain weight, especially the dreaded belly fat, develop insulin resistance that may lead to diabetes, and exhibit high blood pressure. When university students were taken on a three-day forest trip, the amount of cortisol in their saliva decreased 12% just from being present in the forest, and decreased 16% after they walked in the forest. The effect lasted up to a month after their return.

It's interesting to note that a nature experience in a city, for example in a garden, park, or tree-lined path, also seems to increase natural killer cells and decrease cortisol levels in blood. Even looking at pictures of trees can decrease blood pressure and cortisol levels!

In summary, the improvement in immune function and decrease in stress after spending time in nature may be associated with lower rates of infections and cancer, plus less risk of developing chronic diseases like diabetes, heart, and kidney disease.

Researchers in the U.S. and the United Kingdom also cite improved mental function and mood when people spend more time in a natural environment. One study featured 20 people with major depression who took a walk in either a natural or an urban environment. Those who walked surrounded by nature showed a significant improvement in their short-term memory and mood. Ten different British studies involving around 1,200 people found that "green exercise" (exercise in the presence of nature, which is a bit of a loose definition) improves one's self-esteem and mood. People gained even more improvement in self-esteem and mood when there was a body of water in the scenery. Children diagnosed with ADHD show a reduction in symptoms when they spend time in a natural outdoor environment. Researchers continue to investigate the effect of adding nature therapy to prescribed treatment protocols for the disease.

You may know from experience that exercising outdoors, surrounded by majestic trees, lush, colorful plants, alongside a gurgling stream or a sparkling blue lake makes you feel good. But how do you find time in your busy schedule to get away to a forest? If you live in a city, work long hours, or live alone and don't feel safe walking in wilderness by yourself, how can you de-stress your life with nature? We will explore practical ideas and strategies to help you with that in the next section.

Evidence about Nature

1. Parton, J., and Pretty, J. What Is the Best Dose of Nature and Green Exercise For Improving Mental Health? A Multi-Study Analysis. Environ. Sci. Technol. 2010; 44:3947-3955.
2. Berman, M.G., et al. Interacting With Nature Improves Cognition and Affect for Individuals With Depression. J. Affect. Discord. 2012; 140:300-305.
3. New York State Department of Environmental Conservatism. Immerse Yourself in a Forest For Better Health. https://www.dec.ny.gov/lands/90720.html

MAKE IT HAPPEN

Invite Nature into Your Life Even if You Live in a Concrete Canyon

Do you like being outside? Not everyone does. Perhaps you don't like to sweat, or mosquitos find a banquet on your skin, and you'd rather sit in a bar and down dirty martinis. I understand, but encourage you to think about what's at stake. Do you like getting tension headaches every afternoon? Would it be a relief to need fewer medications? How does it feel to toss and turn at night, either when you can't fall asleep, or when you wake up several times in the middle of the night?

Depriving yourself of nature may mean you live in a continuous high-stress state that worsens these and other body ailments. Here are some practices that will help you re-set your body, come down from the adrenaline high of chronic stress and over-stimulation, and enjoy quiet, peaceful natural settings.

- Notice the physical world as you go about your daily schedule.
- When you walk from the parking lot to your school or workplace, do you look at the sky, admire the foliage on nearby trees, relish the soft brush of the wind on your cheek? Between the subway and home, is

there a flower bed where pansies brighten the scene, or a Japanese maple's feathery fronds arch toward the ground? We often stumble through life in an unconscious, unseeing state, dwelling on worries and frustrations and things we need to do. Wake up! It is a beautiful world. If your surroundings offer no natural beauty, then gaze at pictures of trees and sniff essential oils from aromatic evergreens. Studies suggest that even looking at a picture of a tree or forest stimulates activity from the part of the nervous system that lowers blood pressure, relaxes skeletal muscles, and calms breathing. So, find a website (sign in here if you want to view a couple of affirming nature videos I made to keep myself close to nature).

https://stressrelief.deborahrankinrd.com/naturevideos

- Dilute cedar wood essential oil with a carrier oil and dab it onto your wrist (don't use this oil full strength, and avoid it if you are pregnant). Breathe. Take a mini forest break during your day.
- Think about your typical week and select a time when you can spend an hour in a park, along a river or lake, or in a forest. Put it on your calendar, and tell someone about your

> plan to do this. Consider it an appointment as important as anything else in your schedule, and leave your electronic devices behind. Make this weekly time outdoors a ritual.

James Clear wrote in *Atomic Habits* that we should automate good habits, making them automatic choices we do without conscious thought. When we do that, there's no need for "willpower" because our environment makes the good habit a natural choice, and we don't have to make a decision.

I did this one summer when I suffered from chronic vertigo and wished to spend more time in nature to speed my recovery and improve my mood. I was in the habit of going to an early church service every Sunday, and en route passed the entrance to a state park with a lake and six miles of hiking trails. I put hiking boots and clothes in the back of my car, and on my way home from services stopped at the park, changed, and walked a couple of miles around the lake. At first, I felt awkward and clumsy as I walked the trail. The vertigo gave me double vision, and I had to pay close attention to stay on the path and not fall. As I breathed, I imagined mysterious substances in the air filling my lungs with healing molecules. Japanese studies say that when we breathe in forest air, we inhale airborne chemicals called phytoncides that have antibacterial and anti-fungal qualities. I don't know what caused my vertigo, and neither did the neurologist who examined me, but I believe my weekly nature walk helped my recovery. However, I would not have walked there every week if I left it to chance to find a convenient time. Walking became a habit I did without conscious thought, because "it is Sunday, I have my hiking gear in the car, and I always stop to walk when I drive by the park." What will help you make an automatic ritual of outdoor activity?

- Take a weekend detox from work and technology at least once a year. Plan it now. Open your calendar and put a big circle around a weekend within the next month where you will go away to a natural setting. Invite other people only if you know you can spend a weekend together with them in peace and harmony. That might include your spouse or partner. It might not. It might include your best friend, or a brother/sister/cousin. You could take a child that you've been wanting to spend more time with. You could go by yourself. Find a babysitter for the other children, or trade childcare duties with friends. If you tend to put off making travel arrangements (like me), pick a friend or partner who excels at trip planning and sell them on the idea. "Hey! Haven't you been wanting to go to that state park and rent a cabin and fish? Why don't we do it three weeks from now? I'll split the cost if you make the reservations." Whether you sleep in a lodge, tent, cabin,

> or your car, leave your TV and cellphone at home and take to the woods for a weekend. Notice how you feel. Go for hikes, or sit before a campfire and stare at the flames. Row a boat or throw frisbees to your dog. Journal, draw pictures, or color in a coloring book. Breathe.

I've described several ways you can spend more time in nature, from simple daily awareness to a weekly ritual to a scheduled retreat. How will you use this information? What ritual can you build into your schedule to make sure you spend time outside in nature? How can you structure your environment to automate that activity and avoid the need for a decision? Think about this, and get ready to record your next actions on the Key Take Aways and Action Steps page.

BRIAN'S STORY

With more than 1.6 million people squeezed into 23 square miles, the island of Manhattan is six times more densely populated than the soot-smeared, sewage-laden London of Charles Dickens. Surrounded by highways and cut through with taxi- and Uber-filled streets, New York City is not likely the first place to spring to mind when one considers the phrase "getting in touch with nature."

Despite that, you are probably more likely to hear the phrase there than you are to hear it among farmers on the Great Plains or fishermen in Alaska, who are both quite literally in touch with nature and may also see nature as a mundane—if occasionally spectacular—part of daily life rather than some independent end to be sought. But in "the City," the phrase has a particular connotation. For New Yorkers, and wealthy New Yorkers in particular, having a beach house in the Hamptons or a cottage upstate is both a form of spiritual and mental escape from urban life and perhaps more importantly, a symbol of wealth and status.

But what about the person that can't take off "summer Fridays" or long holiday weekends to go to the woods, sunbathe on the beach, or stay in their ski house? What about the person who doesn't have a car and can't escape the concrete jungle without planning ahead and buying an Amtrak ticket or a ride on the Hampton jitney? What does that person do when it feels like the paper-thin walls of their 500-square-foot fourth-floor walk-up apartment are caving in, when the crush of a crowded subway car feels suffocating, or when their eyes burn from spending every daylight hour in the unnatural fluorescent glow of a windowless office?

The secret, if there is one, is to appreciate bits of nature when and where you can. The feel and smell of a softball field in Central Park's Great Lawn is nature, even if you are in the shadow of the three tallest residential buildings in the world and can hear the hum of cars on nearby Fifth Avenue. Nature is the woofs and yips of dogs in Fort Greene Park during pre-dawn or post-dusk "off-leash" hours with the moon rising over Brooklyn Tech's radio tower.

One need not even venture into nature in order to reap its benefits. Finding joy in nature can be observing a hawk perched atop the foul pole during a game at Yankee Stadium, wondering how it has adapted to the cityscape—is it on the lookout for its standard fare, searching for a rodent scurrying somewhere in the concourse below, or is it waiting to pounce when an inattentive spectator drops a hot dog or a chicken tender?

One can find joy in nature by adorning that internal office with a painting of a window looking out into the woods, or by cultivating indoor plants to spruce up the place (so long as you have a friend willing to share some window space from time-to-time).

And an appreciation for nature can come even through the simple practice of meditation. You don't need to own oceanfront property to mentally transport yourself to a lounger on the beach, your toes buried in the warm sand. You don't need a private parking garage downtown to be able to picture yourself deep in the woods on a cool summer night, enveloped by the chatter of squirrels and chirp of crickets.

All you need is yourself, your breath, and your imagination. And a few moments of quiet, if the three roommates you've crammed into your apartment will allow it. Just ask nicely.

—Brian is an attorney who lived in several small apartments during his six years as a resident of New York City. He played in softball leagues that held games in Central Park, and along with his rescue dog Ginger enjoyed the rich social scene of Brooklyn's Fort Greene Park during off-leash hours.

Key Take Aways and Action Steps

Commit to actions you will start now to...

- Cultivate daily awareness of nature.
- Create an automatic weekly ritual of time in nature.
- Plan a weekend get away.

Food, Part 2

FOR IS THERE ANY PRACTICE LESS SELFISH, ANY LABOR LESS ALIENATED, ANY TIME LESS WASTED, THAN PREPARING SOMETHING DELICIOUS AND NOURISHING FOR PEOPLE YOU LOVE?

—Michael Pollan, author and journalism professor

I believe everyone should cook. I believe everyone can cook. Cooking, if planned and organized, takes no more time than ordering a meal and driving to pick it up, or waiting for it to be delivered. The excuse "I don't have time to cook" is, well, an excuse.

You will gain comfort and satisfaction if you learn to cook. To be clear, when I talk about cooking I don't mean baking your own bread or crafting elaborate pastries a la The Great British Bake Off. (Though after watching the show, don't we all now appreciate a proper crumb?) I'm talking about a simple meal you prepare in 30 to 45 minutes, in quantities that leave leftovers for lunch or another weeknight dinner. It's not hard to do. Let's begin by reviewing the benefits of cooking your own meals, then look at some basic principles to follow.

The first benefit of cooking your own meals is that evidence suggest it's easier to achieve goals for healthy eating if you cook at home. Restaurants in the U.S. serve such huge portions that when you eat out you are likely to consume, on average, 200 calories more than when you fix a meal at home. That makes sense given the large portions served in restaurants, the visual appeal of the food, and the tendency to eat more if you dine with other people who are big eaters. Those extra calories, week after week and month after month, increase your odds of gaining weight.

Even though more and more restaurants post nutritional information for their menus and honor special requests, chances are you can fix healthier meals at home. When you do the cooking you also know where the food came from. Is the salmon wild-caught from deep water? It may have a higher content of omega-three fatty acids than farm-raised industrial salmon on a restaurant menu. Were the vegetables grown under conventional or organic methods? What kind of cooking oil is used to prepare the restaurant's fettuccine with sauce: olive oil (unsaturated and heart healthy) or palm oil (saturated and possible to raise your LDL cholesterol)? For those who wish to curtail salt intake to help reduce fluid retention and bloating or lower blood pressure, that is much easier to do with home-cooked foods as most restaurant foods are quite salty. And finally, because fruit perishes rapidly and requires manual labor to prepare, good fruit choices are not common in restaurants. At home, a crisp apple or a bowl of fresh strawberries from the farmer's market are delicious side dishes or snacks. Basic and easy: pick an apple from the bowl on the counter and bite!

The second benefit of cooking at home is that if you cook enough to have leftovers, life is easier because there's always good food around. You are less likely to come home from work hungry, tired, and cranky, and open the fridge or pantry to find nothing good to eat for dinner. Whether you're part of a family or single, it works great to cook only two or three meals a week and plan for leftovers to pack in a lunch or re-purpose into other meals. Let's look at a simple example:

First Meal: Baked chicken, steamed rice, roasted broccoli, and carrots

Second Meal: Leftovers for lunch, re-heated

Third Meal: Chicken stir-fry with peanut sauce, crunchy rice, and orange wedges

Fourth Meal: Chicken burrito with avocado, cheese, and salsa

The third benefit of cooking at home is that it costs less, if you plan ahead and use the groceries you buy. I once heard a physician respond to a patient's claim that she had to eat at fast food restaurants because it was all she could afford.

Their conversation went something like this:

"So, you'll stop off at a fast food restaurant on the way home and buy a Big Meal for you and your mother. How much does one Big Meal cost?"

"Five dollars."

"So for the two of you, you'll spend ten dollars. How much does a big package of chicken thighs cost at the grocery?"

"About six dollars."

"How many thighs in that package?"

"Six or seven."

"You and your mother can have three meals from that one package of chicken. If you buy a bag of rice for two dollars and a bag of carrots for eighty-nine cents, they'll each last for at least three meals. So for a dollar less than one fast-food meal, you and your mother can have three meals at home, with more nutrients and fewer calories, fat, and salt."

The same kind of math holds true for you and me. Home-cooking saves time and money and can yield healthier meals. For parents with children at home, eating meals together is a huge boost to a child's physical, mental, and emotional health. Of course restaurant meals can be shared as a family, but carryout food is often eaten in the car, in front of the TV, or while surfing social media or playing video games. We'll delve deeper into the benefits of family meals in Chapter Nine, "Connect."

For now, what would you and your family gain from cooking more meals at home?

Evidence about Food and Meal Planning

1. Nyguen., B., and Powell, L. The Impact of Restaurant Consumption Among U.S. Adults: Effects on Energy and Nutrient Intakes. Pub Health Nutr J. 2014; 17:2445-2452
2. Junxiu, L., Rehm, C.D., Micha, R., Mozaffarian, D. Quality of Meals Consumed by U.S. Adults at Full-Service and Fast-Food Restaurants, 2003-2016: Persistent Low Quality and Widening Disparities. J Nutr. 2020; nxz299. https://doi.org/10.1093/jn/nxz299
3. Gonzalez, D. The Best Healthy Meal Kit Delivery Services of 2020. https://www.huffpost.com/entry/best-healthy-meal-kit-delivery-services-of-2020_l_5df2b965e4b04bcba180f53b

MAKE IT HAPPEN

Cook at Home and Live to Enjoy It

Cooking is easy, if you have food to cook. While that may sound obvious, creating a habit for buying groceries is the most important action to take if you want to prepare more meals at home. The evening "What's for dinner?" question is not difficult to answer when there is food in the house.

As a registered dietitian and health coach, I advise clients to use one of four convenient ways to make grocery shopping a consistent, weekly habit. It doesn't matter which you choose. Pick a method, start now, and keep it up.

The first is to sign up with the shopping service at your local grocery.

Prepare a standard order, tweak it every now and then for seasonal adjustments, email it in or order online on a set day every week, and pick it up or receive delivery the same day. Voila! Food in the house all week. In 2020, before COVID-19, I surveyed the shopping and delivery services offered by the five largest grocery chains in the U.S. (Kroger, Albertsons, Publix, H-E-B, and Whole Foods.) At that time, fees ranged from $3.95 to free for an online order with curbside pickup. The free options required other commitments such as an Amazon Prime membership or a flat monthly service fee of $14 for Publix. Home delivery cost between $9.95 and $11.95, with no additional charge for those with Amazon Prime or the Publix monthly membership who met a $35 minimum order. Walmart offered free pickup with a $30 minimum order, and delivery costs of $7.95 to $9.95 depending upon order size and location. During the COVID-19 pandemic, to ensure customer safety, almost all grocery chains eliminated the fees for online orders with curbside pickup.

The second method is to use a meal plan kit service. Fill out a profile and a plan for a certain number of meals per week, and receive your food along with recipes and clear directions. This works well for my friend Liz Zorzanello Emery, a single mom, registered dietitian, and Assistant Professor in Nutrition at La Salle University in Philadelphia. Here's what Liz shared with me:

> *I believe in raising independent kids who can be self-sufficient, and am very proud of my girls who are already well on their way in this regard. Last night my 14-year-old son made my dinner. He served cherry balsamic pork chops with roasted broccoli and couscous. I started using Hello Fresh to help with dinner prep while I was working on my doctoral degree. I get a night off, and my son learns to cook - it's a win-win!*

When I had hungry children at home and worked full-time, I couldn't afford a shopping service or meal plan program, so I used a third method. I set aside a certain time every week when I wrote down three or four meals I would prepare that week, made a list of the foods needed for those meals, then went to the grocery! I enjoy grocery shopping, although I understand those who don't may prefer another method for procuring food. When I look at the amazing array of nourishing food choices in American markets, I feel grateful. If I have enough food to eat on a regular basis, I realize how fortunate I am. If you struggle with conflict and guilt over what you eat, return to Chapter Three on journaling, and explore giving thanks for the food options available to you. A mindset shift from food as the enemy to food as nourishment and sustenance can start a powerful life transformation.

The fourth way to make sure you have food in the house is that of the urban walker who stops at a market every day on the walk home from work, subway, or bus stop. My neighbor in Alexandria, Virginia, walks home from his office in Old Town and passes a Trader Joe's blocks from his house. Every day, he stops there and selects foods for dinner that evening. It may not be the most efficient approach, but perhaps it gives him a period of decompression after the rush of a busy work day.

If you find grocery shopping to be stressful, or unpleasant, what can you do to make it a more pleasant ritual? In the essay that follows, Thomas describes how he always puts a favorite food first on the shopping list. Perhaps your market offers free coffee or tea to shoppers, and you can enjoy a coffee break as you shop. I enjoy people watching and am always entertained by the sights I see and the conversations I overhear while shopping. If you choose to shop in person, rather than using a meal prep or shopping service, be present as you shop. Relish the visual panoply of fruit and vegetable colors, converse with the bakers, butchers, and deli staff, and celebrate the goodness of your food supply.

In addition to establishing a consistent grocery shopping method, I recommend buying one fast-cooking device. Just have one that you like and use, so you don't clutter up your kitchen with unused equipment. I am impressed with my Instant Pot pressure cooker. Beef cubes, carrots, potatoes, onions, mushrooms, a can of beer, a sprinkle of spices and a little water turn into a delicious Irish stew in forty-five minutes.

Remember, you don't need to plan a different meal for every day in a week.

You will have leftovers. With basic staples on hand (tortillas, rice, pasta, fresh greens, beans), you can improvise on additional nights and combine leftovers into something new.

If cooking at home is a big change for you, pick a small goal to start. Make it a habit, and make it fun. If you have children in your household, declare that one night a week is make-your-own-pizza night, or pasta night, or pita night.

Stick with it until it's automatic, then do more. Expand your meal planning to cover three family meals. You'll have a night or two of leftovers, and other nights when you'll want to eat out to work around ball games, dance or music classes, etc. If you are single and just cook for yourself, cooking one big meal a week makes an incredible difference. That food, between leftovers and improvised make-overs, can provide dinner meals for up to four days. Leave three evenings open to go out with friends or to treat yourself to a nice restaurant.

Pick a small set of favorite meals and repeat them on a regular schedule so you don't feel pressured to fix something new every week. When my children were young, my goal was to cook four nights a week. I planned one fish meal, one chicken meal, one meatless meal, and one pasta. I had favorite recipes in each of those categories and used them over and over.

By adopting routines, cooking becomes easier and takes less time. Routines protect you from decision fatigue, and establish habits that free your mind. Are you shocked by this basic, repetitive approach? You might ask, "Are you kidding me? You suggest I eat linguini with clam sauce every Tuesday night?" I'm not kidding you. I think that might work quite well. When you eat out, you probably have a certain number of restaurants you frequent over and over. You might order the same thing almost every time you go to a certain establishment. What's different about doing that at home?

If you have children, they love routines.They feel secure as they experience reliability and ritual in the family life. My sons carried the same lunch to school almost every day for twelve years. There were times when I forced them to take something different, or tried to entice them with more creative combinations. Always, they wanted their familiar lunch: One peanut butter and jelly sandwich, cut in half diagonally. A single-serving bag of Cheetos. One apple, cut in half, cored, placed back together and wrapped.

The most touching cooking compliment I have ever received came after a business trip when my middle-school son stayed with a family friend. Apparently he missed my top-notch school lunch. When I returned, he said the sweetest thing: "Mom, nobody makes peanut butter and jelly sandwiches as good as yours."

Dinner for a Slammed Day

Turn the oven to 350.

Take that casserole of pork chops and wild rice from the freezer. Aren't you glad you made an extra serving and froze it when you cooked a couple of weeks ago?

Put it in the oven, then go change into something comfortable. Take the dog/kids/partner to the dog park/playground/bedroom. (Pick only one of the above.)

Have fun.

Come back fifty-five minutes later and pull out a bag of frozen mixed vegetables.

Dump them into a glass bowl, zap in the microwave for two to three minutes.

Remove the bowl of grapes from the fridge.

Put everything on the table and invite your loved ones to dinner.

Talk. Listen. Be grateful.

Dinner for a Typical Day

Come home and look at the list of meals planned for the week.

Linguini with clam sauce? No problem, thirty minutes start to finish.

Boil the water to cook the pasta, fix the sauce, steam some broccoli, and slice a baguette.

"Dinner time!" Wow, that tastes good.

Dinner for an Easy Day

It's cold and rainy, a perfect day for bean soup.

In the morning, pour a one-pound bag of pinto beans into a large saucepan and cover with an inch of water. Let them sit all day.

In the afternoon, pour the beans into a colander to drain the water. (This gets rid of indigestible carbohydrates that give people gas.)

Pour olive oil into a saucepan, chop up one onion, three celery stalks, and two cloves garlic. Saute until soft.

If you eat meat, pull leftover cubes of ham from the freezer and add to the pan along with the drained beans.

Pour water or broth into the pan, add a bay leaf and some dried herbs.

Cover and heat until the combination reaches a gentle simmer.

Fix yourself a drink, if you drink. Sit down in a comfy chair and read a good book.

Look up an hour and a half later. Time to make the corn bread!

Butter a glass pie pan, place it in the oven and turn the oven on to 350 degrees.

Combine one cup flour, one cup cornmeal, 1/4 cup sugar, 1/2 teaspoon salt and 4 teaspoons baking powder.

Whisk together 1 cup milk, 2 eggs, 1/3 cup melted butter or oil.

Add to dry ingredients and stir just until moist. It's OK to leave lumps.

Pour into hot pie pan and cook for twenty minutes. Drizzle local raw honey on top of the hot cornbread.

If you don't like cornbread, you could make quick muffins, or walk to the corner bakery for a fresh ciabatta.

Freeze the rest of the soup for the next rainy day.

THOMAS' STORY

Apples are the first, and most important, item on the list.

I am a person of habit, and perhaps the healthiest and steadiest of my habits is eating an apple as a snack around 10:00 a.m. each day. When my wife Margaret and I make our grocery list for the week, I write apples on the top of the right hand column before even thinking about menus or children's snacks or anything more complex.

Margaret and I anchored our habit of weekly menu planning and grocery shopping while we lived in Paris during graduate school. We were married and close to 30 years old, so we had culinary tastes beyond those of an 18-year-old college student. But we were just as broke as that teenage freshman, living on student loans while paying the mortgage for our house back in Denver. Eating out was not an option, and junk food tended to be more expensive than fresh produce and meat from the weekly farmer's market (you can draw your own conclusions about the respective prices of those items in the U.S.).

So our best option was to methodically plan meals for the entire week and buy only what we could afford on my wife's modest earnings as a 20-hour/week nanny. Lo and behold, that experience became the highlight of our time in France. It drove creativity, as we used seasonal produce and tried to create variety from the same general set of ingredients. It gave us our most natural interactions with French people, like the cheesemonger who teasingly called us "Mister and Missus" in English each week. It brought us together, through the shared time making a shopping list and going to the market. And we ate well while staying within our tiny budget. Perhaps not coincidentally, we were probably in the best shapes of our lives by the end of our time in France.

Nearly a decade later, we still plan menus and buy groceries on a weekly rhythm. I suppose the expected reason for the habit now would be that it creates efficiencies and frees up time and money during our busy lives. We do lead busy lives: I'm the CEO of a growing solar energy company, Margaret is a teacher, and we have three girls under 6 years old.

However, I find menu planning and grocery shopping are not at all about efficiency for me. Rather, they are the times that anchor me, that create peace in chaos. I'll grab a piece of paper and start writing a list after breakfast on Saturday mornings, when the girls are syrup-driven dervishes. I'll "volunteer" to be the one who does grocery shopping, knowing that an hour out of the house with only one girl will be far easier than staying home with the other two daughters. It's a slice of time and life that is positive, under control, restorative, even before we get to making the actual meals.

And I know I'll have my apple each day for the next week.

—Thomas earned degrees in chemistry and energy economics from Washington and Lee University and the Colorado School of Mines. He is CEO of a solar energy company based in Denver. In his spare time, he plays ultimate frisbee, gardens, cures his own bacon and duck breast prosciutto, and enjoys hiking and skiing with his wife and three daughters.

Key Take Aways and Action Steps

What will you do to make buying groceries an automatic behavior? What are three reliable, nutritious, easy meals you can repeat?

Is there a weekly meal ritual you want to establish with your family?

Art

ART ENABLES US TO FIND OURSELVES AND LOSE OURSELVES AT THE SAME TIME.

—Thomas Merton

I grew up in a world devoid of art, in the traditional sense. My family did not go to galleries, buy tickets for the symphony, or take me to the ballet. We went to church. My parents played cards. If I admired poetry, it was that of a basketball player ascending for a rebound, or the couplet of the crack of a ball heading for deep left center and the arc of a bright, swirling orb into the night sky. After a fifth grade field trip to the Museum of Science and Industry in Chicago, I did not enter another large museum until after I graduated college.

A few years ago I went to an art student's senior exhibit at tiny Georgetown College in Kentucky. I stood in the middle of a large white room, gazing at Lennon Michalski's *Ghost Bike*, a motorcycle painted white. I watched a multi-layered neon video of cyclists parading to the graves of lost comrades. I circled the four walls to inspect large, vivid paintings. I spoke to the artist, a slender man so young, so energetic, and probably so relieved to finish his senior project.

As I looked and talked, I realized there was no way I could have done anything like this at his age. I went to college to get a degree that would land a good job with a steady paycheck. For my senior project I designed a nutrition research study in which I created a special chow for caged rats I fed and weighed every day for six weeks.

My parents grew up during the Depression. They got by on what they had and didn't waste money on frivolous things such as art or museums. While they generously provided college educations for me and my three siblings, none of us pursued the liberal arts, even though I always loved to write, and my sisters showed a great aptitude for art and design. We heard the unsaid expectation: "Get a degree, find a job, support yourself."

With such a background, you might wonder why I consider art an important wellness practice. From a dietitian you might expect a formula: eat this many grams of that, exercise this number of reps until you get to this target heart rate, and do this until your cholesterol level goes down to that. Many nutrition and fitness books give formulas. They tempt you with sure-fire promises like "Twenty-Pound Weight Loss in Two Weeks!" and "No More Belly Fat with the Cabbage Cayenne Chocolate Soup Miracle Diet."

If health could be distilled and packaged into a formula, it would have been done and the battle would be already won. Our society would not face rampant rates of diabetes, metabolic syndrome, kidney disease, hypertension, heart disease, and mood disorders.

As humans, we are not only physical specimens. We are body and spirit. Just as our bodies need wholesome, nourishing food, our spirits feed on the transcendent beauty of art. When technology and devices, algorithms and avatars rule our world, art gets pushed out and our spirits starve.

You will improve your health and wellness to the degree that you value and take care of yourself. Art, which in my definition includes the beauty of the natural world as well as the worlds of music, literature, screen, stage, painting, and design, moves your focus from the mundane daily routine to a bigger and brighter vision. When you hear beautiful music, laugh at a comedienne's joke, or admire a painting in a gallery, your spirits rise. You smile, you relax, your breath deepens. Life is good, and you feel good. When you embrace art, and care for yourself by immersing yourself in art on a regular basis, you advance toward the goal of health and wellness.

Although I grew up without institutional art, I spent much of my childhood thrilled by the art of nature. Deprived of symphonies, poetry readings, and art galleries, I enjoyed bright sunny days water skiing on a glassy lake then sitting at the end of a dock dangling my legs in the water as I listened to the peaceful lap of waves against the moorings. I felt the sun warm my face as I stood at the edge of the Grand Canyon. I inhaled damp, sweet, giant redwood air among the sequoias. I recall Disneyland when it was newish, and a southern California that still had orange groves and fresh air. I hiked lush green hills and trod barefoot over smooth rocks in cold mountain streams, then hugged dogs and petted cats and sat on my grandmothers' porches as night fell and cool air drifted up from the creek. I rode bicycles with friends and slid on frozen ponds and skinny-dipped beside dragonflies in the yellow-green water of a rural gravel pit.

Who says what art is, anyway? Is it art if your grandmother crochets a custom sweater for your dog, or your aunt makes a mink collar for your Barbie? What do you call it when your mother presents a hand-made crib quilt at the birth of each of your children? Is it art when your father restores battered desks and tables and turns them into family heirlooms?

More questions, no answers, except I suggest not all art is in a museum.

As an 87-year-old friend of my father wheezed after struggling with his walker up the steps into the church for Dad's funeral, "If I'd known I was going to live this long, I would have taken better care of myself!"

Take care of yourself by making room in your life for art. In the long run, life means so much more than the size of your house, the make of your car, the title by your name, or the dollars in your bank account. While such things may feed your ego, art feeds your spirit.

Decide what represents art to you, then bring it close.

Evidence about Art

1. Stuckey, H.L., and Nobel, J. The Connection Between Art, Healing, and Public Health: A Review of Current Literature. Am J Public Health. 2010; 100:254-263.
2. Hallam, S. The Power of Music: Its Impact on the Intellectual, Social and Personal Development of Young People. Int J Music Educ. 2010; 28:269-289.
3. Kidd, D.C., and Caetano, E. Reading Literary Fiction Improves Theory of Mind. Science. 2013; 342:377-380.

✿ MAKE IT HAPPEN

Nurture Yourself with Art Even If You're Not "Artsy"

Pablo Picasso said, "Every child is an artist. The problem is how to remain an artist once we grow up." If you don't watch out, much of adult life will destroy your instinct and inclination for art.

Read through the following scenarios and circle the one that best describes you.

- You are on a mission to reach your goal. You have a lot to accomplish, and you must get after it. Perhaps you work full-time and go to school at night, or you kick butt at work every single day to prove yourself and get a promotion. You might work more than one job to make ends meet. Art seems like a waste of time and money. You have more important things to do.
- Art? That would be nice, but you're more concerned with getting a meal on the table, making it to the soccer/lacrosse/volleyball games, giving the kids a bath, and helping your parents or grandchildren. You would love to have time for concerts and lectures and book signings. What a great life that

would be! It's just not possible right now. Too many people need you.
- You never really got art. Your parents didn't think much of it, and when you were a kid your mother yelled if you made a tiny splash with your watercolors, or, heaven forbid, dropped a ball of Play-Doh on the floor. And that art teacher in high school! She was weird! And mean. You remember the humiliation when she criticized your drawing in front of the class. You showed her: no more drawing from you.

Even if you have had a difficult relationship with art, it's not too late to learn to enjoy it. But why bother?

Picasso also said, "Art washes from the soul the dust of everyday life." We all get dingy in spirit from time to time, putting up with the same frustrations and challenges day after day, week after week. Art stirs the imagination and takes us to a different place. Through a good book, an entertaining movie, or a beautiful painting, we go to a place where life is fresh and clean. Everything sparkles, or if it doesn't, at least it's gritty and real and makes us feel alive.

While art can wake up our fancies and emotions, it can also calm us. Creating art, or viewing it in a museum, is known to lower levels of the stress hormone cortisol. Listening to music can calm neural activity in the brain, and may help restore effective functioning in the immune system. Scholars say singing has many health benefits, including strengthening the immune system, improving mood, and reducing stress. Multiple studies show that emotional writing, as in journaling, reduces the frequency of physician visits, stabilizes the immune system, and reduces stress hormones and blood pressure. And finally, studies reported in *Science* magazine in 2013 confirmed that reading literary fiction enhanced the ability to understand other people and empathize with them.

Viewing art can help relieve depression and make the world seem brighter. Brain scans show that art triggers release of the feel-good hormone dopamine. I recall a time when I was in a dark and troubled mood before I attended an event at The Phillips Collection in Washington D.C. First, a pianist seated before a glossy black grand piano serenaded us with rippling, cascading waves of beauty. Then guides led us through a special exhibit of paintings by Georgia O'Keeffe. I sucked in the sights of her bright, abstract figures. When I left, I took the beauty of the music and the clarity of the paintings with me. I felt happy. I discovered that taking a break to listen to music and view art reduced my stress and improved my mood.

Make plans to give yourself a gift: make room in your life for art. Get fresh thoughts, reduce stress, and rest your brain. You may discover a way out of a problem that's been bugging you.

For a Slammed Day

This is simple: Art surrounds you, if you look up and notice.

For example, one day at my local Starbucks the service was lethargic. I waited, tapping my foot and checking social media updates every ten seconds.

WHERE IS MY CAPPUCCINO?

HOW LONG DOES IT TAKE TO MAKE A CUP OF COFFEE, ANYWAY?

I imagined a graph of my blood pressure. It arced up into dangerous territory, the red zone marked WARNING!!! In a desperate attempt to calm myself, I looked around. There!

Above the counter where you pick up your order, I saw a captivating photograph. It was big: 3 by 4 feet at least.

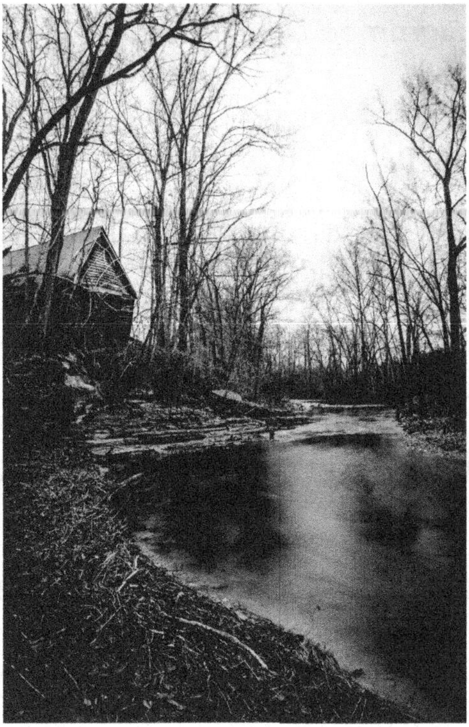

Big East Fork circa 2019. Photograph by David Braud. Used by permission.

I gazed at a riverbank in the country. A rushing stream swept around a bend. Trees extended bare arms toward the other side. I imagined feeling icy cold water when I stepped in. Forces swirled around my ankles, pushing and shoving, but I stood firm, soothed by the current's sweet refrain. The air was fresh and damp. Robins sang.

"Deborah. Tall cappuccino." What? Already?

I took a picture of the photograph with my phone and a man behind me said, “Cool picture. I’ve been here a thousand times and never seen it.”

“Neither have I. Although it was here all the time.” I picked up my coffee and went out to face the day.

For a Typical Day

Option One

The tidying-up guru Marie Kondo says we should look at each possession and ask if it brings joy. Many of us live and work in places cluttered with do-dads that once brought joy, but we’ve tired of them, or our tastes changed.

Today, pick one room of your house and get rid of a thing that does not bring joy. Then pick a painting, piece of pottery, photograph, relic, or textile that delights you. Put it in a prominent space, front and center.

Look at it tomorrow morning as you drink your cold water.

Touch it. Remember where you got it, who made it or gave it to you.

What does it mean to you? Say a prayer of gratitude for that moment, memory, or person.

Not all art costs money or comes from a gallery. My art includes mismatched tea cups I buy at flea markets, greeting cards my granddaughters scribble in bright crayon, a coffee mug embossed with my dead dog's picture, an afghan crocheted by my grandmother, a quilt made by my late mother, one good Navajo rug, and a hand-knotted Persian carpet.

You are the captain of your life. Surround yourself with art you like. Maybe for you it's deer-antler chandeliers.

No problem, I like them, too. Write and tell me where you found yours! For some, a Harley is art. So go to your garage and admire it and dust and polish it. Whatever you do to a Harley.

Option Two

Buy adult coloring books and packs of colored pencils. Stash them in different places for moments of need, such as in your carry on bag when you travel on an airplane, bus, or train. Put on headphones and ignore the person beside you, if you don't feel like talking. Stay calm and happy during long waits on the runway.

You can also keep coloring books in your desk at work. What a great help they are during the fourth video conference of the day! Put up a screen so they can't see what you're doing. Try to appear industrious, as if you are taking notes, but spend the time coloring. Pipe up with a question every twenty minutes or so to let everyone know you're still tuned in.

At home, coloring books can provide relaxation during otherwise-stressful waits such as times on hold to discuss phone or cable TV service or bills, or reviewing claims with an insurance company. I keep them handy for visitors with young children. Everyone likes to color!

For a Light Day

This is when you plan your next art outing. Strive for a fun art activity at least once a month. Whether you go to a concert, book signing, movie, or gallery opening, be intentional and schedule something you've been "meaning to do."

Ask friends to go, buy tickets, put it on your calendar. Hire a babysitter if you need to. Trade off with friends if you can't afford a sitter. Won't that be fun? Now you have something to look forward to.

SANDY'S STORY

I work very hard as the editor of the poetry journal *Rockvale Review* and the director of the Rockvale Writers' Colony. My days are busy and varied; my responsibilities range from reading submissions to designing writing workshops and advertising promotions to pulling weeds in the garden and mopping floors. I love what I do, even when the 12-hour days roll one week into the next, but I'd be lying if I said it wasn't stressful. At times, I feel like my head is so stuffed with responsibilities that one more might make it explode.

There are a few things that counter the weight of that responsibility for me. Playing the piano is one. Being outside in nature is one. Art is another. It's hard to explain how the visual comforts the visceral, but it does. Maybe it's fascination, or appreciation, or just plain awe, but art books, art museums, even art pages on Facebook calm me, lower my heart rate, and set my busy mind at ease. I have multiple books on artists, complete with photos of their work: Winslow Homer, Vincent van Gogh, Mary Cassatt, Auguste Renoir, Gustave Caillebotte, Edouard Manet, Edward Hopper, and more. I devour these books.

Reading them and gazing at the art helps me forget my problems and stressors. I pay attention to the artist's skill, style, and subject matter. I dive deep into their world, into the images that haunt them, and find myself out of my own world and into theirs. Maybe that's the key. Creative, imaginative people find comfort in creativity and imagination. Visual learners find comfort in the visual—things they perceive as beautiful and meaningful.

I've taken it a step further, though. I create visual art myself: mixed media, watercolors, acrylic pours. Art days are play days, times when I set my "Director" hat in the closet, pull my hair back into a ponytail, throw on an old T-shirt, and get elbow-deep in paint. Although it's not mindless, it feels that way.

Although there is structure, it feels risk-free. I'm not afraid of making a mistake, of scraping paint into the trash can if I don't like how it looks. Nothing is permanent. Even a dried canvas can be painted over. Art days are times for experimenting, for trying something brand new when success doesn't matter, when exploration is the key and the purpose.

It has an effect on me I can only describe as magical. I'm light, almost floating, in stress-free creating. The stress I carried from work is somehow broken up into pieces, carried out on the breeze. I forget who I am in the official sense and recognize myself in the heart sense – as a Creative, as an Artist. I hold that feeling inside me when I return to work, and I'm renewed, inspired to think deeper and out of the box, to let my imagination take over when I face the paperwork, the planning, the accounting, the correspondence. What used to be a coil of stress is now a river of possibility. What used to be just another day of work is now a day of potential that I can make as beautiful as my creativity allows it to be.

—Sandy Coomer is an accomplished poet whose publications include three chapbooks and one full-length poetry collection. She founded and edits *Rockvale Review* (rockvalereview.com), an online poetry journal that publishes two issues a year. The journal presents poetry by established, emerging, and beginner poets and pairs each poem with a piece of art or photography chosen by a featured artist. In 2018, she followed her passion to support and encourage writers of all genres and career stages and established Rockvale Writers' Colony (rockvalewriterscolony.org), a safe, comfortable, and inspiring environment in rural College Grove, Tennessee, where writers work on projects during week-long residencies or attend themed weekend retreats. In addition to her artistic pursuits, Sandy is an endurance athlete, completing a full Ironman triathlon and competing in the 2017 Ironman 70.3 World Championship race. Follow her at sandycoomer.com

Key Take Aways and Action Steps

Write down your thoughts about what art means to you and the kind of art that stirs your soul and calms your mood. Then, when you're ready, make a commitment to:

- Mindfully notice the beauty of the world around you.
- Highlight artistic beauty in your surroundings.
- Schedule an art outing.

Exercise

EXERCISE IS A CELEBRATION OF WHAT YOUR BODY CAN DO. NOT A PUNISHMENT FOR WHAT YOU ATE.

—Anonymous

I began my video book review of John Ratey's book *Spark: The Revolutionary New Science of Exercise and the Brain* with this rhetorical question: https://deborahrankinrd.com/spark/

"If there was one pill that could lift depression, improve the reading scores of dyslexic children, raise school performance, calm people with ADHD, blunt the cravings of an addict, and slow the process of aging, would people take it?"

I think we know the answer. I could add: "If I had a secret sauce that gave you more energy, helped you accomplish more at work, made you feel happy, drained stress, maintained your brain function as you aged, and helped you sleep better, would you want it?"

Of course you would.

I know that secret sauce! I'll help you discover it! The secret is...(drum roll, please)

Move your body.

The benefits of exercise are so mind-blowing, I don't understand why we all aren't exercise enthusiasts. You would go nuts for any other treatment that accomplished what exercise does. You would buy it and not care how much it cost.

Unfortunately, many of you have paid for fitness in the past yet not received these promised benefits. Is there a treadmill collecting dust in your basement? Do unused bicycles clutter your garage? And the gym membership—is there an automatic charge on your credit card every month, but no sweaty workout clothes in your laundry basket?

Multitudes of research studies tell the ways exercise keeps your body and mind healthy. I will reference a few studies later in this chapter, but here's a quick overview of what exercise can do for you. Exercise helps you:

- preserve lean muscle as you age
- sleep better
- feel less depressed
- lower your risk of heart disease, kidney disease, cancer, and diabetes
- achieve better blood sugar control, for those with diabetes
- improve balance
- increase mental alertness
- maintain mental function
- reduce headaches and back aches
- handle the challenges of travel

Exercise helps you FEEL GOOD! Feeling good is its own reward. When you approach exercise with that perspective, it ceases to be a punishment, a burden, something you have to do. When you love moving your body, it becomes a habit you want to do! It is how you live. It might help you lose weight, but more likely it will help you keep off any weight you lose. Exercise conquers the struggle with your weight.

The U.S. Department of Health and Human Services recommends 2-1/2 hours of moderate aerobic activity a week, coupled with muscle-strengthening activity two days a week. Brisk walking or fast dancing count as moderate activities. Muscle-strengthening activities include lifting weights or doing pushups or planks. To me, the details of how many minutes you exercise are not as important as starting where you are, and improving. If you've been inactive for years, beginning with a ten-minute walk in the morning and a ten-minute walk in the evening is a huge step forward. If you do that consistently, you'll get a health boost.

Entrepreneurs and creative artists experience depression and burnout at rates higher than the general population. Whether this stems from the high expectations, individual responsibility, and unrelenting pressure of the work, exercise is a proven way to reduce the severity and side effects of depression and burnout. An analysis published in 2018 found that resistance exercise training was associated with a significant drop in depression symptoms: lifting weights twice a week led to an improvement on par with taking anti-depressant medications. The online version of *Entrepreneur* magazine declared that regular exercise helps entrepreneurs become more confident, creative, and energetic leaders. "Being an entrepreneur is one of the most stressful jobs, and regular exercise helps entrepreneurs unwind and be prepared to face the challenges of the next day." A 2018 article in *Forbes* stated exercise was "the single most important habit for achieving super success."

Even more exciting, walking improves creativity and the ability to come up with new ideas. While walking either indoors or out both enhance the generation of new ideas, walking outside seems to produce the most novel and high quality thoughts. Stressed entrepreneurs seeking solutions to complex customer needs, and creative artists who need to form something meaningful and beautiful from the wisps of their imaginations, will find that regular exercise sharpens their minds.

In summary, regular exercise can improve your mental function, learning ability, medical conditions, mood, and work success. Exercise helps you be the best version of you. It unleashes your energy and creativity. Next, we'll discuss simple and effective ways to make exercise a consistent and pleasurable part of your life.

Evidence about Exercise:

1. Ratey, J.J. With Hagerman, E. Spark: The Revolutionary New Science of Exercise and the Brain. New York: Little, Brown and Company; 2008.
2. bit.ly/DeborahRankinreadsSpark

3. Gordon, B.R., McDowell, C.P., Hallgren, M., Meyer, J.D., Lyons, M., Herring, M.P. Association of Resistance Exercise Training With Depressive Symptoms: Meta-analysis and Meta-regression Analysis of Randomized Clinical Trials. JAMA Psychiatry. 2018; 75:566-576.
4. Pandiata, R. How Fitness Can Ensure a Smooth Entrepreneurial Journey. Entrepreneur.com 1/7/2019.
5. Cohen, J. The Single Most Important Habit For Achieving Super Success. Forbes.com 10/19/2018.
6. Oppezzo, M., and Schwartz, D.L. Give Your Idea Some Legs: The Positive Effect of Walking on Creative Thinking. J Exp Psychol: Learning, Memory and Cognition. 2014; 40:11424-1152.

MAKE IT HAPPEN

Learn to Enjoy Moving Your Body

To forge a path for improving your fitness, let's start with a few questions about your feelings about exercise. From the options below, circle the statement that best describes you:

1. I know I should exercise. I do when I have time. I'm just not consistent.
2. I hate to sweat. I've never worked out. Gyms are yucky and I would not be caught dead wearing skin tight workout clothes in a room full of strangers. Exercise is just not my thing.
3. I love to exercise, but I've slacked off recently due to [broken foot, injured knee, achy joints, other illnesses].
4. I probably would exercise if I knew a good way to start. I'm scared to just show up at a gym or class, and I can't afford a personal trainer right now.
5. I am on it. I've got this one nailed.

The approach that will work best for you to develop a regular exercise habit depends on how you feel about working out. Read the suggestion that aligns with your selection above.

1. You exercise sporadically, when you remember, and have time.

Any activity crammed into leftover scraps of time is not going to be a game-changer. If this is your situation, you may have months of inactivity for every week or two in which you embrace a new fitness plan (like the first two weeks of January, or the month before your beach vacation or high school reunion). You take one step forward, two steps back. Are you a victim of Big Step Syndrome?

Big Step Syndrome is when you believe health and wellness require a total, drastic makeover. It stems from a voice inside that says, "You aren't making it. You need to get your act together and change! Everything!" In the past, you probably embarked on heroic ventures: you implemented a 1000-calorie or Adkins or juice diet at the same time you started running five miles a day or joined a boot camp program. You are bold and courageous to take Big Steps. I applaud you. Yet the sad truth is that your huge commitment and heroic effort often don't succeed because the body's internal defense mechanisms interfere.

Behavioral scientists say the human brain resists big changes. Change brings unfamiliar experiences that the mind views as a threat. To protect yourself, your subconscious mind resists by creating excuses, distractions, or self-doubt. These creations derail compliance with the Big Step, and you return to your prior habits.

You are more likely to affect lasting change if you adopt small, simple behaviors and make them automatic so you don't even think about them. No decision is required; no willpower is needed. It is just what you do. We've discussed this approach for other areas of health such as eating breakfast, sleep, and meal planning. It works for exercise, too.

Knowing that the best way to lock in a good habit is to make it impossible not to do, here are examples I've seen work well for clients or colleagues:

- Co-workers call each other at noon every Monday, Wednesday, and Friday. "Let's do it." They walk two laps around the company parking lot, a distance of about a mile. Because they do it together, they keep each other accountable. A side benefit is the opportunity to share juicy corporate scuttlebutt when pals can talk freely, away from prying ears in the cubicle corral!
- A busy working mom brings her toddler home from day care, grabs the stroller, water bottle, and dog's leash from the handy place where she keeps them stashed inside the back door. She takes her child and the dog for a walk around the block before doing anything else. After a few days, it's a habit. It is very hard for her to overcome pressure from the child and the dog because both insist it's time for their walk!

- A homeowner cancels the lawn service and begins to mow his own lawn with a push mower. This is a good aerobic workout, and with headphones and the roar of the mower surrounding him, he gets away from all the people in his life who hassle him. Mowing the yard becomes his personal escape, a mini-retreat. He has always been fanatical about his lawn. Without a landscaper on retainer, there is no way he'll skip lawn mowing. He can't let his yard get out of shape!

If your exercise history tends toward on-again off-again, the best way to build a consistent exercise habit is to pick something small and doable and make it automatic.

2. You have never worked out, and left to your own devices, you never will.

It's hard to adopt a behavior you've never done before, which means you need help in the form of a coach or mentor. That's OK, it's good to ask for help. Why struggle alone to learn something when it is easier with a guide?

I think of my friend Cindi, a dear person I've known for more than twenty-five years. Cindi is a hard-working and successful corporate executive who demonstrates great artistry and skill in her personal life. She is so artistic she can flip through a swatch of paint colors three inches thick, rustle them back and forth, then pull out one and say "That's it. Paint your wall this color." The color always looks perfect. Cindi can host a dinner for thirty people without breaking a sweat, and fix eggs benedict for a group before I finish drinking my first cup of morning tea.

She is a gifted woman, but she is not an athlete. During the years we've been friends, I've encouraged and invited her to exercise. Twice, I pushed her to exercise. Once she rollerbladed with me, but her face got so red after two hundred yards, I feared she would have a stroke and begged her to stop.

Another time, she attended a restorative yoga class with my encouragement and developed horrible hemorrhoids that required surgery. Still, I know she lives with high stress due to the demands of her job, and I want her to experience the calming effects of exercise. Finally, I told her I knew she had never exercised in her adult life, I understood she hated to sweat, and I remembered several good efforts she'd made like the rollerblading, the yoga, in addition to the expensive rowing machine that now collected dust in her attic. I suggested she find a guide, a personal trainer, and encouraged her to look for a small gym, with a knowledgeable trainer who could teach her how to work out. We talked about how important it was for her to take care of herself, because her body's strength was essential if she wanted her career success to continue. She should spend money on her body, just as she spent money on her hair, nails, and clothes.

I give Cindi credit. She found a personal trainer in her neighborhood. You can read how that worked for her in this chapter's essay, "Cindi's Story."

When life crushes you, when you have tried and failed, or when you've failed to try, a coach and guide make a difference. It is a worthwhile investment at any stage of life.

My father became depressed after my mom died and he lived alone for the first time in his eighty years. The solitary winter days seemed dark and dreary. Since my brother is a physician, Dad listened to my brother's medical advice:

"Studies show that weight training is good for senior citizens. If you work out, you will sleep better, keep your blood sugar under control, get better balance, and reduce your risk of falls and fractures." My brother, bless his heart, gave more than advice. He gifted Dad a three-month package with a personal trainer at a small local gym.

My dad lived seven more years after Mom died. That gym membership made his life worth living, and turned him from lonely to lively. He had a routine. He went to the gym every Monday, Wednesday, and Friday at 8:30 a.m. He became acquainted with others who worked out then and made new friends. He got strong, and he liked to show off how easily he could lift his suitcases when he traveled. He became an exercise evangelist and recruited other senior gentlemen to start working out, too!

After three months of working with a trainer once a week, my dad continued the workouts on his own. He kept it up for the rest of his life, and life was better for him because he exercised. At age eighty-seven, with cancer in his soft tissue and brain, when we went to the funeral home together to plan his memorial services, he proudly and confidently walked up the middle of the twenty concrete steps into the funeral home without needing to hold a railing for support. Although cancer got him, exercise gave him more life in his years. I believe working with a trainer helped him do this.

3. You love exercise but somehow got out of the habit.

Your life situation changed, and you forgot to alter your exercise habits in response. Even though you enjoy working out and have been very good about it in the past, what used to work isn't feasible now. This is not unusual. Life changes, and we forget to adjust our workout plans to the new scenario. Can you no longer run because of nagging knee or hip pain? Try TRX, rowing, bicycling, swimming. Did you drop out of your tennis league because you travel more for work? Get some headphones, build a workout playlist, and de-stress after a hectic day on the road with walk and run intervals on the hotel treadmill. The kids' schedules are more demanding, and there's no time for two-hour hikes or bike rides on weekends? Join a spin studio and compress your workout into a shorter time, or get up an hour earlier and do three thirty-minute high-intensity workouts a week before you go to work. Experiment with a jump rope or weighted hula hoop.

When I broke a small bone in my foot and couldn't walk or bicycle for two months, I took private Pilates sessions to learn how to modify movements and protect my injured foot. Then I bought a series of group Pilates classes that featured a reformer, a cool device I loved. I discovered a new type of workout I'd never tried before and developed core strength I had long needed!

If you look at your life situation with a fresh eye, discerning what workout ritual fits best, you can navigate a life transition with ease if you create a new exercise routine to match a change in lifestyle.

4. You're willing to exercise, but don't know how to go about it and can't afford a personal trainer right now.

Never fear, many types of movement bring significant health benefits but don't cost much. Don't be a victim of Big Step Syndrome. You don't have to join a gym, hire a trainer, or invest thousands of dollars in new equipment.

The most basic exercise of all is walking. You can walk at home; you can walk as you commute to work or catch a commuter bus, train, or subway; you can walk in your work location at lunchtime or climb stairs or walk to speak to a colleague in person rather than talk on the phone; you can walk in a shopping mall or health club or take laps around the field and gym as your children practice sports; you can walk on a treadmill while watching the news or your favorite TV program. Regardless of your circumstances, chances are you have an opportunity to walk. Depending on the condition of your knees, hips, and back, however, before you begin a walking program it might be worth spending $80 to $100 on a good pair of walking shoes. I go to running stores where the clerks are trained to watch me walk and help me find the shoes best for my feet and gait. Plan to buy new walking shoes every three to six months, or about every 500 miles walked. Although I don't keep track of my miles walked, I always notice that my knees or hips often start to ache when my shoes get old. That signals me to toss them and buy a new pair.

Another low-cost, easy way to break into exercising could be classes offered at your public library, community center, or parks. Many community swimming pools offer free or low-cost water aerobic classes. One public library I frequented offered phenomenal free yoga classes every other Saturday. Classes at free venues such as these are often not extremely intense. Other students and teachers tend to be welcoming and helpful. If you are intimidated by the idea of joining a gym, class, or boot camp program, you might enjoy starting slow with free classes that boost your confidence while you build your fitness.

Public libraries also offer exercise videos and DVDs for checkout, while a plethora of fitness instructors publish YouTube videos of their classes. The success of this approach depends on your personal inclinations. I personally don't enjoy exercising at home with a fitness video. I am energized by being around people, enjoy the personalized attention and adjustments I get from a skilled instructor, and become bored exercising to a video. Yet I'd bookmarked one yoga instructor whose hatha exercise video helped me release deep muscle tension, and I found it a wonderful resource when COVID-19 made it impossible to go to class. Overall, though, I do better working out outside, inspired by the beauty of nature, with friends or groups, or in conjunction from a distance with other people. Be realistic about what works for you: Is it likely working out alone with a video is a habit you will keep up? Is this a habit you will stick with?

We all go through times when money is tight and you need to find free workouts. However, our human nature places a lesser value on anything free. Spending money represents a commitment that may strengthen your resolve to keep at it. If you have had little success in the past sticking to exercise, free programs may not the best for you. If you hire a trainer, buy passes to a class, or pay for membership to an exercise club, you will probably see better results.

5. You have a regular exercise habit that you enjoy.

Congratulations! Keep up the good work. Now, see what happens when you integrate exercise with other core habits of wellness, such as journaling about how exercise enhances your life, observing the beauty of nature as you exercise, or combining exercise with art by listening to music or gazing at art while you workout.

If you struggle with injuries or nagging aches and pain from your exercise, go multi-sport and alternate different types of activities.

Quotes to consider:

Ten minutes a day of movement is better than none. If you have never exercised, start small and keep it up.

Find an activity you enjoy.

Lifting weights twice a week led to a remission rate for depression on par with taking anti-depressant medication.

Exercise is a way to take care of yourself.

It is a gift you give to YOU.

CINDI'S STORY

When I was a child, it seemed like the adults in my life either hit me or begged me to eat. My mentally ill father abused me physically, and I was sickly and frail. In tenth grade, I developed mononucleosis followed by Epstein-Barr Syndrome. The disease persisted for over a year, and I required a home-bound teacher because I was too weak to attend school. I was hospitalized with toxic shock syndrome at age 17, and it took me another year to regain strength. I got married at 19, moved to a new location, and felt healthier until I needed surgery to clear a pelvic abscess after the birth of my second child.

For the next 15 years, I went from doctor to doctor, trying to understand why I didn't feel well. My early physicians prescribed anti-depressants. As a normal person given anti-depressants, I went into a fog and became depressed. I lived that way for 15 years. It was awful. Often I wanted to leave my family and get on a bus and start over somewhere else. I felt they would be better off without me. I could not hold down a job because I missed so much work from illness.

When I worked all day I came home and went straight to bed because I was so exhausted I couldn't function. I was given drugs to sleep, drugs to stay awake, and drugs for anxiety. I took medications for high cholesterol and high triglycerides. I was on loads of medications and I was only in my twenties and thirties!

When I turned 40 and weighed over 200 pounds, a friend referred me to her physician. After many tests, he said I was severely hormone deprived and needed to detox by weaning off the many medications I took. I planned to start a new job in three months and wanted to be able to work the long hours required. With better medical support, I met that goal. During a year of detox, I followed a vegetarian, no sugar diet, and lost thirty-five pounds. I felt like a new person.

Soon I took a job in outside sales and soared. I was promoted and traveled widely for work. I traveled for ten years and was promoted twice more. With each promotion came more stress. I knew I needed to deal with that but I never seemed to have the time.

Finally, I decided it was time to exercise. I joined a neighbor with a home training business. My workout buddy was 76 and our trainer was 70. I went twice a week for two hours and it wore me out at first. Two months after I started working out, I was diagnosed with type 2 diabetes. I was devastated! I began medication and planned to take it only until I got my diet in check. A year later I was still on medication for diabetes and could not get my HbA1c into the desired range with diet alone. Although my training was interrupted when complications from an earlier ruptured appendix necessitated hernia repair, I recovered for two months and started training again.

After two years of exercise, I lost 30 more pounds and feel stronger and happier than I have in years. People tell me I look great. It is a journey, but I love it.

During the COVID-19 pandemic I could not exercise with my buds but plan to resume. I have a rowing machine I use at home and I started walking again. At 57 I began a new career and I want to work for ten more years.

If I can get in shape after all of these years, YOU can, too. My husband says he is proud of me. He continually compliments my dedication and hard work.

Recently, as we dressed for an event, I was looking at the back of my hair with a mirror, and yelled to him, "Something is wrong with my back! I've got lumps. Please come look."

He came over, looked, and said, "You have muscles! That's what they look like. They are defined, versus the fat you used to have."

It was really funny because I've never had anything like that on my body before. When I shave my legs now it takes longer, as they are more round. More new muscles! I tell people I used to be a marshmallow and now have hard spots.

I love my exercise routine. It's a journey. I am ever-evolving!

—Cindi is a sales executive with a national supply company. She enjoys life with her workout buddies, husband, children, and grandchildren. In retirement she aims to help women boost their esteem and confidence through proper body wear. Learn more at www.myessentialbodywear.com/A13205.

Key Take Aways and Action Steps

Spend time writing how you feel about exercise, and brainstorm a list of actions that would be practical and doable small steps for you. Pick one.

Work

A CULTURE THAT FUNNELS ITS DREAMS OF SELF-ACTUALIZATION INTO SALARIED JOBS IS SETTING ITSELF UP FOR COLLECTIVE ANXIETY, MASS DISAPPOINTMENT, AND INEVITABLE BURNOUT.

—Derek Thompson, writer at *The Atlantic*,
NPR commentator, and podcast host

Economists and thought leaders early in the 20th century claimed automation and technology would shorten our work week so much that deciding what to do with all our leisure time would be a huge issue. In fact, according to Thompson, today the most affluent and educated among us now have less leisure time and work longer than those in the middle and lower income classes. He says it's because of the religion of workism: "the belief that work is not only necessary to economic production, but also the centerpiece of one's identity and life's purpose."

Getting a handle on your expectations about work is critical for your health.

While health and fitness are vital for your long-term career success, as we discussed in the last chapter, you will find it difficult to dedicate time to your health if you expect your job to provide all your identity and meaning.

Most of us struggle with the balance between cultivating our careers and honing our health. I have been the hard-working, ambitious, and successful professional who felt tired, overwhelmed, and burned-out. I know what it feels like to juggle car, rent, or mortgage payments, pay off college bills, and rear children while aiming for success at work or trying to find a better job. Anyone reading this book can likely recall occasions when you felt drained, burned out, or trapped.

About ten years ago I felt stuck. I fantasized about quitting my job, selling everything I owned, and absconding to a small beach town where I would live in a tiny cottage and support myself by waitressing in a diner near the beach. That appealed to me because when I looked ahead in my current situation, I saw a long slog to retirement. I didn't want to endure life, crossing off weeks, months, and years until I could do something more satisfying. I felt trapped by my respectable, moderate success.

Because of that experience, I began this book with the idea that work was part of the problem. I planned to use my perspective as a health coach, wellness advocate, and nutritionist to help readers focus more on healthy habits. I did not plan to write about work. When I shared my chapter topics with trusted advisors, one said I needed a chapter on work. "We spend a lot of time there. It's an important part of our lives."

Wow. I realized we do spend a lot of time working, thus an absence of boundaries with work can be a big obstacle to our health goals. I wondered if I needed a new mindset about work: one that didn't view it as either a necessary evil to endure, or the source of all life's purpose and meaning. What if work is just the place where we exercise our skills and gifts in a useful way, and in return receive resources on which to live? Is it possible to do that kind of work without sacrificing one's physical and mental health?

I think so. Here is a checklist to help you assess how well your work fits you.

- Does it support and align with your core values?

One of my core values is that food gives life—physical life, emotional life, spiritual life. Over a 40-year career I've held a huge variety of jobs, but most were somehow related to food. No matter how much or how little money I earned, whether I loved or hated my boss, when I did work that aligned with that value I felt a purpose that kept me strong and healthy. During the years when I fantasized about waitressing at the beach, I made more money than at any other time of my life, but my work had nothing to do with food. It did not align with that core value, but read on. In the **Make It Happen** section, I write about the importance of keeping an eye on the big picture, and tell how my lucrative but unfulfilling job did support another core value.

- Does your work put you near people you admire and respect?

If you work around top-caliber people, you'll learn much from them. You'll feel inspired, even if your job is routine and otherwise unrewarding. If those you emulate are replaced by others less sterling, as often happens in the corporate world (my internal cynic quipped in the past that good bosses come and go, but bad ones hang around forever!), then you have an opportunity to rise up and become an example and role model yourself. Just remember that the traits of those you spend time with seep into you. If you sense you're falling to their level, get out.

> *If you run with wolves, you will learn how to howl. If you associate with eagles, you will learn how to soar.*
>
> *—Colin Powell, retired four-star Army general, Chairman of the Joint Chiefs of Staff, and 65th U.S. Secretary of State*

> *Who we are and who we become is in large part the combinatorial product of the people we surround ourselves with—what William Gibson so memorably termed our "personal micro-culture" and Brian Eno called "scenius."*
>
> *—Maria Popova, writer and art commentator known for her blog Brain Pickings*

- Is it time to reassess?

A career lasts a long time—40 years if you are lucky. It's a good practice to step back and ask yourself at regular intervals if it is time to give yourself permission to try something different and veer from the expected path. Make the best decision you can with the information you have at the time. Hang on to a sense of humor. I faced a big career decision 20 years ago when presented with a good opportunity that required me to leave a role as a health care professional I had enjoyed for over 15 years. Did I want to become a business person? I wasn't sure. One afternoon I sat in a co-worker's office and flipped a coin. Heads meant stay, tails meant go. I took a deep breath, said a prayer and tossed. It was tails. "Eh. Maybe I'll do two out of three." I flipped the coin three times. It landed on tails every time! Although I was uncertain about leaving a career I loved, I took the new position and discovered it fit my personality and style in a way I had not expected. I kept that coin. When times in the corporate world got crazy, I looked at the coin and remembered to keep an open mind. I was only there because of a coin toss! So set aside occasional time out of your routine, perhaps in a planning retreat or personal year-end review, to look within and consider if it is time for you to move in a new direction.

- Are you holding back from an opportunity because you fear failure?

Work is a big part of life, but remember it is not your life. You have value and worth, no matter what happens at work. If you go all out for success, there will be times when you fail. When that happens, don't despair. Get up and keep moving.

> *Success is not final, failure is not fatal: it is the courage to continue that counts.*
>
> *—Winston Churchill*

I like work. I'm not afraid to tackle big jobs or daunting circumstances, and through good bosses and excellent opportunities I've been blessed with upward mobility and increasing responsibilities. Even so, I've experienced setbacks and failures. During one hard time in my career I faced three disasters in quick succession: My beloved father died after an ugly battle with cancer, my job was cut during a corporate merger, and I developed chronic vertigo and double vision. I was grieving, jobless, and sick.

I did not work for two years after those calamities. I tried to find a job. I networked, honed my elevator pitch, updated my resume many times, and applied for 287 jobs, but I did not get one job offer. I felt hopeless and lonely. Several long-time friends abandoned me.

A quirky series of events finally led to a job offer. A job-seeking buddy told me about a Chamber of Commerce ribbon-cutting for a new business that had the word "Cabernet" in its name. We often went to chamber events together to network. This time, we went because we thought we'd get a free glass of wine. Imagine our disappointment when we discovered that the business hosted painting classes. There was no wine, free or otherwise. Yet, at this event my pal introduced me to the corporate recruiter who eventually placed me in a job.

I felt healthier once I was back at work. Having a purpose and routine is good, and the healthiest people are often those who keep "working" their entire lives, either in paid work, a family business, or as a volunteer. Yet I grew a lot as a person during my furlough from work and developed new skills I'm happy to have now.

While it's good to do work that aligns with your values and interests, the common advice to simply "follow your passion" does not guarantee success. Business writers such as Jim Collins, author of *Good to Great*, and Jeff Goins, author of *The Art of Work*, say a better approach is to look for the sweet spot where talent, opportunity, and passion intersect.

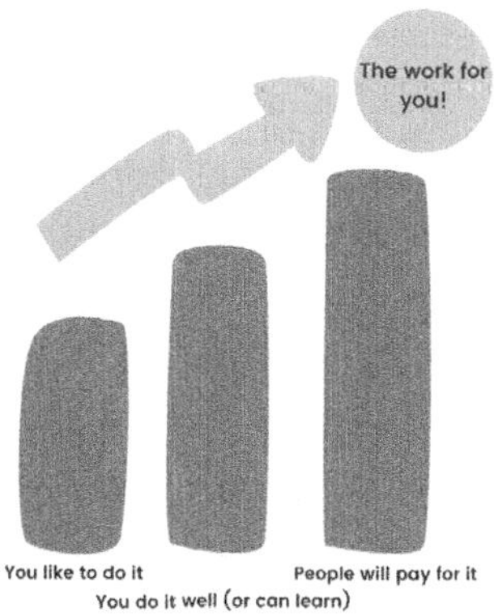
The work for you!
You like to do it
People will pay for it
You do it well (or can learn)

That means seek something you like to do, something you are good at doing, and something people will pay good money for you to do. Even when it's something you like to do, there will be moments of tedium. Perhaps not every minute Yo-Yo Ma practices the cello is sublime, yet he retains the joy of playing. Mr. Rogers discussed the importance of enjoying what you do in an interview with Charlie Rose:

> Families have written to us and said their kids wanted to learn the cello...because they saw on the program how much [Yo-Yo Ma] loved his work. If adults can show what they love in front of kids, there'll be some child who says, 'I'd like to be like that!' or 'I'd like to do that!' said Fred Rogers. He told a story about a sculptor in a nursery school he was working in when he was getting his master's degree in child development: There was a man who would come every week to sculpt in front of the kids. The director said, 'I don't want you to teach sculpting, I want you to do what you do and love it in front of the children.' During that year, clay was never used more imaginatively, before or after. A great gift of any adult to a child, it seems to me, is to love what you do in front of the child. Because you know, attitudes are caught, not taught.

Find a purpose, work with people you respect, reassess every now and then if it's time to change, try again when things don't work out like you hoped. Enjoy each day, and you'll de-stress your life with work that matters.

Evidence about Work

1. Thompson, D. Workism Is Making Americans Miserable. The Atlantic, 2/24/19.
2. Popova, M. Oliver Sacks on Storytelling, the Curious Psychology of Writing, and What His Poet Friend Taught Him About the Nature of Creativity. https://www.brainpickings.org/2015/06/19/oliver-sacks-thom-gunn-writing/
3. Goins, J. The Art of Work A Proven Path to Discovering What You Were Meant To Do. Nashville: Harper Collins; 2015.
4. Hamilton, D.R. Why Kindness is Good for You. London: Hay House UK; 2010.

✿ MAKE IT HAPPEN

Keep Your Eye on the Big Picture

Have you ever asked yourself why you work? Perhaps the answer seems obvious. You work to pay rent or mortgage, buy groceries, save for retirement, and maintain health insurance. You may see work as a practical necessity, without an inspiring or life-changing purpose. Is there anything wrong with that?

During the period when I fantasized about chucking everything and moving to the beach, I led a team selling office supplies and lived in a state with a low cost of living. I earned more money and had more disposable income than I had at any other point in my life, but I felt stifled because my job wasn't interesting or life-saving. We sold office supplies! I supervised tedious and boring tasks like updating huge contract spreadsheets with thousands of line items for thousands of customers. I saw no uplifting purpose in my work.

Then my son got sick. Because I could afford a beautiful home with a pool in a serene, park-like neighborhood, I gave him a restful refuge where he stayed for weeks and recovered. Then my father got sick, and because I'd moved closer to him for this job, I visited him most weekends and helped him arrange his affairs as he approached the end of life. Through this lucrative but tedious job, I provided for two people I cherished. Did my job have purpose? Yes. It honored another of my core values: families support and nurture each other.

As Dad was dying, the company announced plans to merge with another. I had considered filing for family medical leave, but with the merger looming I kept working so I could do my best to help my employees keep their jobs. Then I got a pink slip weeks after his death.

All this is to say it is not easy to decide how much devotion to give your work. No one has the perfect answer. If someone tells you they have the answer and knows exactly what you should do, run from them! I find comfort in advice my dad wrote in a letter for me to read after his death. He told me some things related to handling his affairs, then ended with these memorable words:

> *Things may get a bit messy.*
> *Just do the best you can.*
>
> *—Roger Thomas Rankin*

The best you can do is listen to your gut, do your best at the job you have, and persevere regardless of the obstacles and challenges you face. A career lasts a long time. If you contribute top-quality work every day and demonstrate honesty and integrity, you will recover from any missteps to soar higher and brighter than before. Don't let your job ruin your life, and also don't get confused and think your job IS your life. Thrive somewhere in between! Let me share practical approaches that help me find balance between my work and my personal life.

- Always take all your vacation time. This is so obvious I feel foolish saying it. It seems absurd to think there are people who don't take all their vacation, but I've heard there are. Don't be one of those people.
- Don't work on weekends, unless you are in a field like health care, hospitality, real estate, or law enforcement, where serving people on weekends is part of the deal you signed up for. If your responsibility or workload is such that it's impossible to take the whole weekend off, then dedicate at minimum one entire weekend day with no work. In the Scriptures, God prescribed a day of rest each week. It's a healthy practice. I don't work weekends, so I always feel refreshed and energetic on Monday morning, with new inspiration for the week ahead.
- Keep separate devices for work and personal use. I made that iron-clad rule after I worked for a boss with no boundaries. She worked every weekend, and habitually emailed at 6:30 Saturday night or 7:00 Sunday morning. The tipping point was a Christmas Eve when I picked up an email with a question about a contract, and instructions to resolve it in two days, as I rode a chairlift to the

top of a ski mountain in Colorado. I have learned that if I have a work device with me on weekends and vacations, I don't have the willpower to stop checking email. When I read about work, I start thinking about it. I lose a vacation's rest. Know yourself, and do what you need to do to disconnect on weekends and holidays. Since I know myself, I've kept separate work and personal devices for years. I turn off my work phone and computer at 5:30 Friday evening and put them in a cupboard where I can't see them.

- Create a ritual that signals when work is over for the day. That is especially important when you work from home. Without a ritual to end work, the work day never ends. Establish a cue that tells your body it is quitting time. It could be a song you play, a pair of jeans or shoes you change into, or an activity with your child or dog. When I had a dog, I signaled the end of the work day by clipping on her leash and going for a walk. I relaxed and got in a happy mood.

We each have purposes to accomplish on this earth. Work is an honorable endeavor that channels our skills so we make a difference, even if it's as mundane as finding and correcting an error in a spreadsheet. More than once in my career, a job I disliked because it was low level or paid less than I thought I deserved was the exact place where I learned wonderful new skills that positioned me for an amazing new opportunity. At work, we forge partnerships with others, accumulate resources for our future, and develop new expertise.

There will be tough times. Here are practical steps for reducing stress during different types of work days.

For a Slammed Day

The best approach for crazy days when disasters come at you like heat-seeking missiles is to relax. Don't resist.

Notice, and let yourself feel it as you say, "Wow. This is a really bad day."

Admit it, and go with the flow. Then...

- Hydrate. Drink eight ounces of water at morning, noon, and the end of the work day.
- Walk up and down a few flights of stairs if your health and fitness level allow.
- Look at pictures of forests, as recommended in the Nature chapter.
- Put harsh emails in your drafts folder and wait until morning before sending them. Re-read then, and decide if that is still the approach you want to take.

- Find a person who is struggling and say a kind word, make a joke, or just smile at them. Kindness stimulates the release of a hormone called oxytocin, which causes the release of nitric oxide in your blood vessels. Nitric oxide expands the blood vessels and reduces blood pressure. Choosing kindness amid craziness helps YOU feel better!

For a Typical Day

Think about the 80/20 rule. Of everything you might do today, what drives results? Do that.

If you work in a highly virtual or digital environment, make time to speak to someone. Ask them what they did this weekend. Do they have a team in the big game? The gel of human connection cushions us from life's bumps and potholes.

If you work in a location with others, get up from your chair once an hour and walk down the hallway or around the room.

Before you leave for the day, make a short list (no bigger than a Post-it note) of what you want to accomplish tomorrow.

For a Light Day

Call or send an article to your mentor.

Get involved with mentorship if you're not already. Check in or share an inspiring quote with your mentee.

Use the extra time to both give and receive.

Review your projects, client list, and programs. Determine the revenue or impact of each and re-calibrate based on which ones are in your 20%. What are your goals for them? How can you strengthen your relationships with those colleagues or clients?

Take a step in that direction.

Read a newsletter, white paper, or magazine related to your work. Re-charge and refresh with new ideas.

Express gratitude for three things you like about your work.

MEGHAN'S STORY

My name is Meghan, and I am a lover of food, wine, books, yoga, swimming, and outdoor activity. I am also a registered dietitian in New York City and a recovering workaholic. Paradoxically, my obsession with becoming a "health expert" made me stressed, tired, and unhappy.

My journey to earn the registered dietitian credential was not an easy one. When I started graduate school, I worked two jobs, volunteered at a hospital twice a week, and commuted two hours into New York City for class three nights a week. I got home around 11 p.m. each night and woke up at 4:30 the next morning to exercise. I had no social life.

I kept that type of schedule for almost three years. I was physically exhausted by the time I began my dietetic internship in the Bronx, and my passion for nutrition was waning. I knew this lifestyle was unsustainable, but I had no idea how to break away from it. One day I read an article about the importance of self-care (for a school assignment, ironically), and came across a quote by Michelle Obama:

> *We need to do a better job putting ourselves higher on our own 'to-do' list.*
>
> *—Michelle Obama, two-term First Lady and podcast host*

This seemed like a simple idea, but it shocked me. I realized I had been the lowest thing on my to-do list for years. During my primary care rotation at the hospital, I worked with a wholistic dietitian who incorporated stress management, yoga, and meditation into her nutrition education programs. In addition to diet recommendations, she encouraged each of her patients to schedule 30 minutes of self-care time daily. Remarkably, the patients that fully integrated themselves into her whole health program kept coming back to the clinic and seemed happier and more equipped to manage their health conditions.

Research shows that stress is associated with high blood pressure, heart disease, and weight gain. And yet I was completely uninformed about this as a dietitian-in-training. It was not easy for me, but I realized I needed to force myself to take time away from work. I started small: a walk during my lunch break every day and one yoga class per week. These small commitments sparked a transformation in my approach to work-life balance.

There is much pressure to be successful in today's world, often at the expense of our health. People are rewarded for staying at work late and pushing themselves to the point of exhaustion to get ahead. After years of struggling with work-balance myself, and working with patients who have health issues related to this type of lifestyle, I now understand that our bodies need breaks.

Today, I make every effort to leave work on time. I try to avoid checking emails outside of work hours. I still take walks during lunch. I make regular plans to see family and friends. Since I have not allowed my job to take over my life, I enjoy going into work every day. Most importantly, I feel healthier than ever.

—Meghan Donnelly is a registered dietitian based in New York City. She earned a Master's degree in Nutrition & Dietetics from New York University and completed her clinical training at the Bronx VA Medical Center. Her nutrition specialties include weight management, digestive health, and kidney disease. You can find out more at www.nutmegnutrition.org

Key Take Aways and Action Steps

As you reflect on this chapter, ask yourself:

- What information about work was new to you?
- How well does your work align with your core values?
- When was the last time you assessed your work and life objectives?

Connect

"IT IS BETTER TO EAT TWINKIES WITH GOOD FRIENDS THAN TO EAT BROCCOLI ALONE."

—John Ortberg, theologian and author

The Alameda County Study tracked 7,000 people over nine years and found that the most isolated people were three times more likely to die than those with strong connections with other people. People who smoked, had poor diets, were obese, or drank too much but had strong social ties lived significantly longer than people with great health habits who were isolated. Harvard researcher Robert Putnam said if you belong to no groups but decide to join one, you cut your risk of dying over the next year in half.

During the last 50 years, the American way of live shifted due to social changes like more frequent moves and relocations, shorter tenure in jobs, a higher divorce rate followed by more adults living alone, longer work hours, and fewer in-person interactions as a result of increased use of technology. While many of us understand we can improve our health by eating better, exercising, stopping smoking, and staying sober,

I'm not sure we grasp how important it is to have good connections with other people.

Here are relevant quotes that illustrate the importance of strong interpersonal connections:

- Loneliness is as dangerous to your health as smoking, and a bigger risk than obesity and a sedentary lifestyle.
- Prolonged social isolation carries the same health risks as smoking 15 cigarettes a day.
- Twenty-two percent of American adults report they often feel lonely, and lack companionship.
- Generation Z (adults age 22 or less) are the loneliest age group.
- Greater social connections are associated with a fifty percent reduction in the risk of early death.

These are not tabloid headlines. Respected researchers, leading universities, and government agencies base these alarming conclusions on sound scientific information.

I feel sad when I read these studies. I mourn for the elderly widower sitting alone in his house day after day, for the young adult holed up in an apartment with hundreds of channels and thousands of Instagram followers but no one with whom to share a pizza on Friday night.

I worry about myself, too. I've always worked long hours, and for eight years I traveled for business at least half of each month. That made it hard to make friends and difficult to stay close to my current friends when I'm not always available to join activities. Like many Americans who work for large corporations, I've moved every three to five years and must start over to build friendships in each new town. I've lived alone since a divorce almost 20 years ago. Do these loneliness factors negate my health efforts? I wonder.

I believe the ideas emphasized in this book are vital for strength, health, and quality of life: nutritious food, enough sleep, a journal, art and nature, and meaningful work. Since wellness involves the whole person, however, personal connections deserve our attention, too. I wrote this chapter on personal connections to remind us that wellness is not just a formula to adopt in a New Year's resolution, for example, "I am going to give up all sugar." Do I think it's healthy to eat less sugar? Yes. Have I cut my sugar intake more than I ever expected I would be able to? Yes. Yet if I want true health I need to keep my heart open to other people, and make room for them in my life. After a long day's work, when I'm tired and tempted to hibernate at home in front of the TV instead of going to an event or joining friends, I remind myself:

> *Social isolation is as strong a risk factor for disease and death as sedentary lifestyle, high blood pressure, smoking, or obesity.*

This is a hard chapter to write because the topic seems so...obvious. Does anyone want to be lonely? Of course not. Then why are we? Frayed family ties, geographic mobility, a high divorce rate, long work hours, substance abuse, and addiction to technology are just a few things that separate us from other people. Reconnecting can be as simple as sharing family meals, joining a local organization, or going to church.

When I mention loneliness, perhaps you picture a solitary person alone in front of a TV. You can also be lonely if you live with others in parallel lives that don't include much real connection. With separate cars, TVs in bedrooms, and heads buried in devices, a family can live in the same house without often connecting with each other. One report says the average number of family dinners in a week dropped a third between 1981 and 1997, and another says that 60% of the time when we eat together, TV or technology or an outside form of entertainment joins the meal as a distraction.

Sharing a meal with another person is an act of connection and emotional intimacy. It requires that we set aside other activities to face one another. We reach out for food, we give sustenance to others. By stopping the work, putting down the book and the device, and ignoring the calls and texts and emails we say, "I am here, in the present. I see you here, too." It is the pause and the presence that enables connection. When we smile, tell funny stories, share a small insignificant detail that might never come out otherwise, we feel known. We sense "someone heard me." Even when dinners are loud and raucous, when children fight and spill milk, perhaps one brother dares another to fling ketchup on the wallpaper or incites outrage by grabbing the last French fry, a shared meal gives a physical connection that says "I am real, I belong, this is my place."

Psychologists and sociologists produce many studies about the benefits of family meals for children, as do non-profits like The National Center on Addiction and Substance Abuse at Columbia University and The Family Dinner Project. When I read their reports, I begin to think a parent could do a lot of things wrong but still raise sound, healthy children if they just ate meals together about five times a week! Family meals are associated with many benefits: better academic performance, higher self-esteem and more resilience, lower rates of alcohol and drug use, less risk of depression, less obesity, fewer teen pregnancies, eating disorders, and suicides. Of course it's not just the act of eating together that binds us, but the interaction that occurs around the dinner table. Academics at Emory University's Center for Myth and Ritual in America Life say dinnertime conversations increase family knowledge, adjustment, and resilience. When we retell family legends, rework the narrative to explain and clarify, a child develops perspective, critical thinking, and a knowledge of her role within the family. The single strongest predictor of high academic achievement and low rate of behavioral problems for children is home-based family meal time.

In his book *Bowling Alone*, Robert Putnam said social connections within America started to decline in the 1970s and continued to fall off into the present because of pressures of money and time, mobility and sprawl, television, and generational differences in relating. I remember when life was different. My father-in-law worked hard, but he was home for dinner almost every evening at five. I know a man from my hometown who has played on the same church softball team for over 50 years! I can't report such a stable schedule or long-time involvement with a group, and I expect most of my readers can't either.

We humans are social animals. Just because we have enough money to live alone or to live with someone in a house with a big lawn set back from the street where the neighbors' noise and quirks will not intrude, it doesn't mean peace and quiet is all we need. Bored, depressed, restless, lethargic? Perhaps you need deeper social connections. Join an organization, club, or group. Beautify public spaces with the garden club, ride with the Harley club instead of by yourself, take your dog to the dog park and start a conversation with another dog lover. Going to church is another way to connect with people, and in fact there is a solid body of evidence confirming the benefits of church going.

Researchers in northern California began to study residents of Alameda County, California, in 1965 to investigate the relationship between lifestyle and health. As they followed over 5,000 people, collecting questionnaires, blood values, and health reports between

1965 to 1999, they identified five lifestyle choices that improve health:

- Stop smoking
- Exercise regularly
- Maintain a healthy body weight
- Sleep seven to eight hours a night
- Limit alcohol consumption

These are well known now, so accepted they seem obvious. In the sixties, however, smoking, inactivity and drinking were not big worries. The Alameda County data paved the way for "new" approaches like smoking cessation programs, the running craze of the seventies, and Jane Fonda's aerobics classes in the eighties.

In 1997, researchers used the same Alameda County data to evaluate the relationship between church attendance and health. Based on 28 years of follow-up, they found that people who attended religious services once a week or more had a lower mortality rate. Frequent church attenders were also more likely to stop smoking and increase exercising, stay married to the same person, and have more social contacts. These associated lifestyle factors would be expected to improve health and reduce mortality on their own, yet the association with religiosity and mortality remained even when the other factors were taken into account.

More recently, in 2017, researchers from Vanderbilt, UCLA, the University of Mississippi, and Charles Drew University School of Medicine used data from a big government-sponsored study called NHANES III to look at stress levels, attendance at religious services, and mortality in adults between the ages of 40 and 65. They found religious service attendance was linked with lower mortality, even when adjusted for difference in education, income, and the presence or absence of health insurance. More frequent attenders had a 55% lower mortality rate! In this report there was no "dose-response" effect of going to church—those who went once a month had a drop in mortality similar to those who went once a week. Church attenders seemed to have less metabolic stress, as determined by health markers like blood pressure, cholesterol levels, laboratory markers of inflammation like homocysteine and C-reactive protein, waist-hip ratio and hemoglobin A1c, a marker for blood sugar control among those with diabetes. The authors commented that the health benefits of active faith might be attributed in part to compassion and a sense of holiness deriving from active, personal faith. Compassion creates a sense of generosity and unselfish concern for others that helps us cope with stressful situations as we find a greater connection with those around us. They said holiness gives meaning and purpose to life, and instills love, joy, peace, and hope through a personal relationship with a higher power.

This is fascinating data, but I would not want anyone to attend religious services for the health benefits alone. God is not a cosmic bellhop I manipulate to achieve things I want by placating with certain behaviors. Regardless of how or why religious attendance helps one's health, I mention the studies for several reasons. First, they surprised me: I had never heard of them until I started my research for this book. Second, the ideas are evidence-based, drawn from established databases and published by academic professionals in peer-reviewed medical journals. Many popular health and diet trends have far less scientific validation. Third, they align with the central theme of this book: health and wellness involve the whole person.

When you get frustrated with your weight or your fitness or your appearance, it is tempting to latch onto a simple formula espoused by the latest guru or internet personality. That person convinces you "If I just give up___________ or take up __________for ___________days/weeks/months I will never again have to worry about _____________." We all want the magic bullet, the quick and easy solution.

I am here to tell you there is no magic bullet, no simple formula that will change everything. There are small, daily habits you build into your life by making them automatic so you don't have to think about them. Since distances between us are greater, particularly in the post-COVID-19 world, forming habits of connection with other people is just as important a health practice as exercising and eating nourishing food.

Health may be the greatest resource you have: in the end, health is more valuable than the amount of money in your 401k, and all the money in your portfolio may not be able to buy health once you lose it.

Healthy habits are not tortures you must endure to get a trimmer figure or better results on medical tests.

Healthy habits are their own reward. Good food, enough sleep, expressing yourself in a journal, using your time wisely, celebrating nature and art, exercising, and connecting with other people work together to generate energy and vigor and release stress. They help you feel better and enjoy life more.

You can do it. De-stress your life. Turn chaos into calm.

Evidence about Connection

1. Ortberg, J. Everybody's Normal Till You Get to Know Them. Grand Rapids: Zondervan; 2014.
2. Housman, J., and Dorman, S. The Alameda County Study: A Systemic, Chronological Review. Am J Health Education. 2005; 36:302-308.
3. Holt-Lunstad, J., Smith, T.B. Social Relationships and Mortality Risk: A Meta-analytic Review. PLoS Med. 2020 July; 7(7): e10000316.
4. The Importance of Family Dinner VI. The National Center on Addiction and Substance Abuse at Columbia University, 2010. https:// www.centeronaddiction.org/addiction-research/reports/importance-of-family-dinners
5. The Family Dinner Project, a non-profit initiative started in 2010. Massachusetts General Hospital Psychiatry Academy, Boston. https:// www.thefamilydinnerproject.org

6. Duke, M.P., Fivush, R., Lazarus, A., Bohanek, J. Of Ketchup and Kin: Dinnertime Conversations as a Major Source of Family Knowledge, Family Adjustment, and Family Resilience. The Emory Center for Myth and Ritual in American Life. Working Paper No. 26, May 2003.
7. Putnam, R.D. Bowling Alone: The Collapse and Revival of American Community. New York: Simon and Schuster; 2000.
8. Doherty, W.J. Share the Table: The State of Dinnertime in America. A White Paper Study Published by Strategy One, a Daniel J. Edelman Company.
9. Strawbridge, W.J., Cohen, R., Shema, S.J., Kaplan, G.A. Frequent Attendance at Religious Services and Mortality over 28 Years. Am J Pub Health. 1997; 87:957-961.
10. Bruce, M.A., Martins, D., Duru, K., Beech, B.M. Church Attendance, Allostatic Load and Mortality in Middle Aged Adults. PLoS ONE 12(5):e0177618

MAKE IT HAPPEN

Build a Network of Support

Now that we've established social isolation as a credible health risk, what will you do? Perhaps you set goals to lose weight or vow to run a marathon, but do you think about building healthier relationships? Do you believe that's important? I learned the hard way to nourish my emotional and social needs so isolation and loneliness don't affect my health.

I consider myself a strong, healthy person. Through most of my life I've been blessed with good health. A few years ago I went through a horrible, awful, very bad year when my beloved father died, I was laid off from my job, and a long-time friend abandoned me in a heart-breaking way. Within months, I got a chronic case of vertigo and developed high blood pressure. At the time, I felt like I was cursed: getting sick seemed like just one more way in which life or fate or the powers-that-be conspired to make me miserable. Now I suspect these conditions were at least partially related to my extreme stress and the loneliness I felt when I lost so many important connections in a short time.

People vary in how much social connection they need and want. You know if you're more of an introvert or an extrovert. Yet social connection is not a matter of whether you more enjoy a cocktail party with a hundred new people or a quiet walk with an old friend. It is who do you talk to, and how often... do you have people who know what's going on in your life? Is someone there for you when the bottom falls out? How many people know what matters to you? Do you share activities together?

Reading is a solitary activity favored by introverts, but many readers enjoy a book club. Hikers can be quiet, reflective people, yet travel together to hiking destinations. Introverted beekeepers like my brother attend workshops and conferences and relish talking with honey aficionados at the farmer's market every Saturday. Writers join critique groups.

Because social connection is such a personal, individualized factor, instead of giving specific action items for how to make it happen, as I have done in previous-chapters, I will ask you to meditate on four statements and what they mean for your health:

- Social connection is a fundamental part of a healthy lifestyle.
- Doctors in the United Kingdom now write prescriptions for structured social activity. Do you need one?
- A recent study of 20,000 adults by Cigna found that those age 22 years and less had the lowest social engagement of any age group. If you know a young adult of this age group, is there an activity you could take up together?

- If you want more friends, be a friend.

I struggle with social isolation myself because I live alone, work long hours, and for much of life have lived many miles away from my family. A few months ago I remembered how important are my friends when I faced what I made into a health crisis. (In reality, it was quite minor.)

I have good teeth and have needed only one filling in my entire life. That cavity was filled back in the dark ages of my youth when the dentist used a giant syringe with a horrendous long needle and a drill that shook the whole building with a raucous grinding sound. Recently, this ancient filling came loose and needed replacement. I was petrified. I could think of nothing else for days. I couldn't focus on work. The back of my neck was tied in knots. The morning before this "massive operation" I texted three friends and asked them to pray for me. Yes, pray for me, over a filling! I am sure both they and God had more important business at hand. But bless their hearts, they responded with encouraging words, compassion, and concern. They supported me, and I survived. Although perhaps I remained tense, because several times during the quick and painless procedure the dentist told me to remember to breathe.

From this situation I realized good social connections are about having someone to call when you're terrified about a tiny little filling, to whoop and holler with you when you win the big deal, and to cry or curse with you when you don't. It's someone to stand beside you on the sidewalk when you buy concert tickets from scalpers in the no-scalper zone, and to talk with on the phone for hours on a long drive so you don't fall asleep at the wheel. It's the person who tells you when you have lipstick on your teeth, and the one who lets you use their address when you want to stay incognito. A friend is someone who knows who you really are, and likes you anyway.

Treat your social connections with the same importance you give to whether you eat sugar or Paleo or 5/2 fast or do cardio or weight training. You are a whole person. The National Wellness Institute says there are emotional, occupational, physical, social, intellectual, and spiritual domains to wellness. Through healthy connections with other people you gain strength and healing in all six domains.

TERRY'S STORY

What is it about sharing time, thoughts, and hearts over a cup of coffee or a meal that grounds and centers us? How is it that through such conversations and sharing we find out more about ourselves than we do the others?

One of the blessings of living a creative life is being surrounded by other creative hearts. And, as any of those who've enjoyed my creative workshops or retreats will tell you, my philosophy is that all hearts are creative if we just believe and act on that belief.

However, in most cases, living a creative life requires solitude in order to create. If we are not careful, writers, photographers, and the like can become isolated. For me, isolation can be restorative in small doses but draining over time. I need the give and take of the energies of others to re-energize.

Flannery O'Connor said, "I write because I don't know what I think until I read what I say." A lot of times, I don't really know what I think until I share it in conversations with others. Then magic happens as they respond. I find that even in disagreement, there are threads of agreement, and my thoughts change and improve.

As we share and interact with others, connections arise. They are not created, for they were always there. They arise as we give them life through our engagement. The connections bring us the energy, validation, and love from other hearts, all carried in the grace of genuine listening, sharing, and caring.

When we visit and share in person, we follow new paths that lead to deeper levels of understanding of both the other and of ourselves.

The root of the terms communication, community, and communion comes from the Latin communionem, meaning "fellowship, mutual participation, and a sharing." Communion is typically associated with the sharing of sacraments in a religious worship. However, we often refer to sharing of meals together as a form of communion, a time that also leads to a sharing of lives and of hearts. A communion at church is a community ritual experience of symbols of sacrifice. A communion of hearts involves a sacrificing of egos in favor of a deeper vulnerability—an opening, if you will, of the small, sacred spaces within—that perhaps even we have not explored.

It is in the discovery and unearthing of those small, sacred spaces that we can begin to live from them. It is from those spaces that we become intimately acquainted with our authentic self, embrace it, and live from it.

Living from our authentic space pushes us to create from that vulnerable place. Creating from our vulnerable place compels us to recognize others who are striving to do the same. And that results in a transcendent extending of grace to the other.

And in one of the beautiful, alchemical moments of life, it is in the extending of grace to others that we learn to embrace it in ourselves and become involved in, as poet, priest, and philosopher John O'Donohue wrote, the "difficult spiritual work of learning to love yourself."

The journey of loving others and ourselves is where healing starts. How amazing to think all of this can begin over a good cup of coffee or meal.

—Terry Price is a writer, photographer, labyrinth facilitator and retreat leader who lives on a farm near Nashville, Tennessee, with his wife and three dogs. He enjoys spending lots of time with the four perfect grandchildren who come to visit. Learn more about his work at www.terryprice.net

Key Take Aways and Action Steps

What tiny threat, such as my new dental filling, reminded you that you need help and support from others?

How can you make connection with other people a higher priority? Who do you want to get closer to?

Helpful Tools

Things to Check Out

- Ujjayi breath is a kind of controlled breathing used in yoga, particularly in the vinyasa or hatha styles. There are many online videos that demonstrate ujjayi breathing, but I prefer to work with a local instructor to get personalized direction whenever I start any new yoga practice. However, I found this article to be helpful as a description and overview of the benefits of ujjayi breath.

  https://chopra.com/articles/learn-the-ujjayi-breath-an-ancient-yogic-breathing-technique

- While essential oils add much sensory pleasure and relaxation to my life, it's important to learn how to use them safely. Consult with an experienced guide before proceeding, and always store essential oils in a secure area out of the reach of children. Here's a helpful guide to safe use of essential oils, including lists of those that increase sun sensitivity, and those that should always be diluted with a carrier oil before applying to your skin: www.doterra.com/US/en/essential-oil-safety

- Berry, W. *The Selected Poems of Wendell Berry*. Berkely: Counterpoint Press; 1999. Your local independent bookstore can order this book for you, or it can be purchased from Amazon.
- Want to know if you have habits that may lead you to burnout? Take my free quiz to look for signs of stress in your life, and then decide your best course of action. https://deborahrankinrd.com/view-burnout-quiz/
- David Braud is the photographer featured in the Art chapter. Find more about his work at davidbraud.com

Acknowledgments

Many people helped and encouraged me as I wrote this book.

First I want to thank my sons and daughters-in-law who listened to my ideas with infinite patience. In particular, thank you Thomas for suggesting the work chapter, Margaret for encouraging me to return to my roots and write about nutrition, Brian for your input on the Make It Happen section, and Karen for helping form the title.

The eight people who contributed essays for the book so generously shared their wisdom. In addition to Thomas and Brian, thank you Stephanie Hsiang, Amy Millican, Sandy Coomer, Cindi Rutledge, Meghan Donnelly, and Terry Price. I am deeply grateful for your contribution! I encourage readers who'd like more information about their businesses or products to follow them via the links in the biographical paragraph that follows each essay.

Two wonderful and wise people served as beta readers and gave valuable feedback! Thank you, Mike Duncan and Julie Williams.

My dietitian mentor Sohailla Digsby guided me on this path and helped set deadlines so I finished the book.

Always, ever: Mom and Dad. Gone but not forgotten. Thank you for the years of fresh garden vegetables, home cooking, and strong connections with your families and friends.

Made in United States
North Haven, CT
20 October 2026

20740133R00114